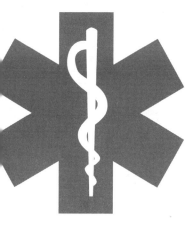

Pediatric Case Studies for the Paramedic

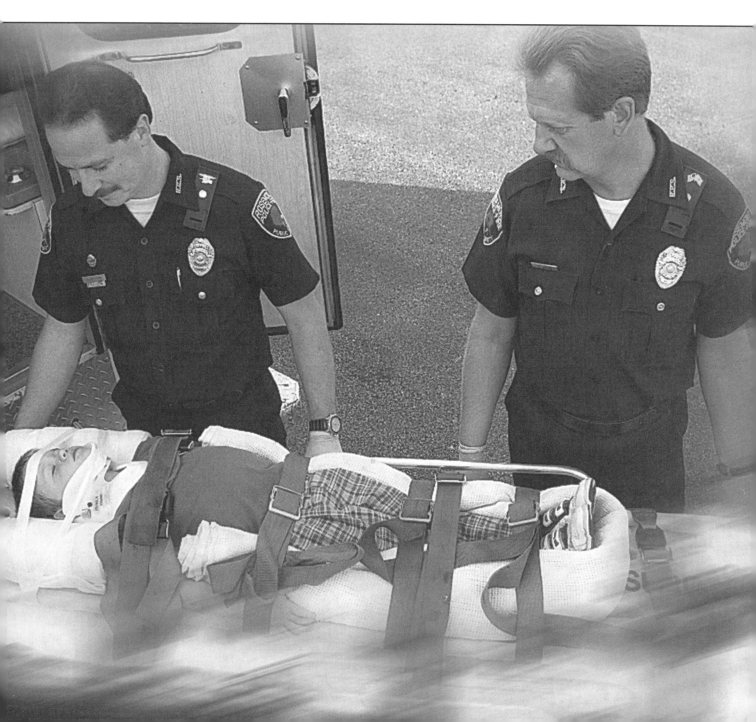

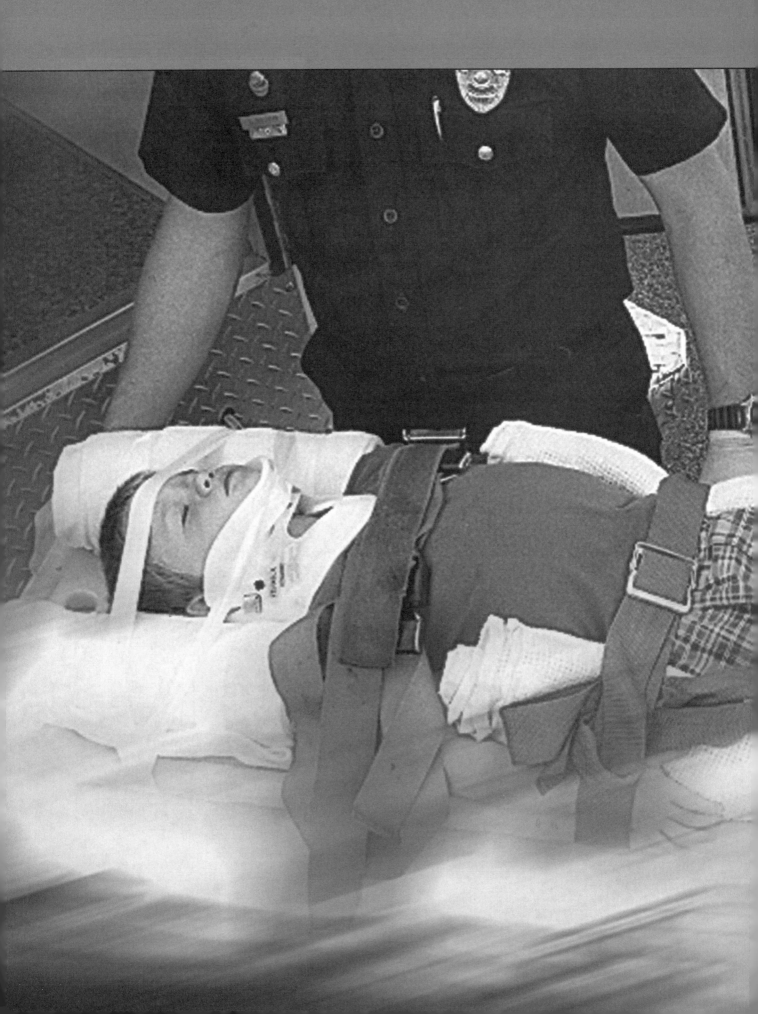

Pediatric Case Studies for the Paramedic

Stephen J. Rahm, NREMT-P
EMS Professions Educator
Bulverde-Spring Branch EMS
Spring Branch, Texas

Andrew N. Pollack, MD, EMT-P, FAAOS
Medical Editor
University of Maryland School of Medicine
Baltimore, Maryland

JONES AND BARTLETT PUBLISHERS
Sudbury, Massachusetts
BOSTON   TORONTO   LONDON   SINGAPORE

World Headquarters

Jones and Bartlett Publishers
40 Tall Pine Drive
Sudbury, MA 01776
978-443-5000
info@jbpub.com
www.EMSzone.com

Jones and Bartlett Publishers Canada
6339 Ormindale Way
Mississauga, Ontario L5V 1J2
Canada

Jones and Bartlett Publishers International
Barb House, Barb Mews
London W6 7PA
United Kingdom

American Academy of Orthopaedic Surgeons

Editorial Credits

Chief Education Officer: Mark W. Wieting
Director, Department of Publications: Marilyn L. Fox, PhD
Managing Editor: Barbara A. Scotese

Production Credits

Chief Executive Officer: Clayton Jones
Chief Operating Officer: Donald W. Jones, Jr.
President, Higher Education and Professional Publishing: Robert Holland
V.P., Sales and Marketing: William J. Kane
V.P., Production and Design: Anne Spencer
V.P., Manufacturing and Inventory Control: Therese Connell
Publisher, Public Safety: Kim Brophy

Publisher, Emergency Care: Lawrence D. Newell
Associate Editor: Janet Morris
Production Editor: Susan Schultz
Text and Cover Design: Anne Spencer
Composition: Jason Miranda, Spoke and Wheel
Cover Photograph: © Jones and Bartlett Publishers. Courtesy of MIEMSS
Printing and Binding: Courier Stoughton

Jones and Bartlett's books and products are available through most bookstores and online booksellers. To contact Jones and Bartlett Publishers directly, call 800-832-0034, fax 978-443-8000, or visit our website, www.jbpub.com.

Substantial discounts on bulk quantities of Jones and Bartlett's publications are available to corporations, professional associations, and other qualified organizations. For details and specific discount information, contact the special sales department at Jones and Bartlett via the above contact information or send an email to specialsales@jbpub.com.

This manual is intended solely as a guide to the appropriate procedures to be employed when rendering emergency care to the sick and injured. It is not intended as a statement of the standards of care required in any particular situation, because circumstances and the patient's physical condition can vary widely from one emergency to another. Nor is it intended that this textbook shall in any way advise emergency personnel concerning legal authority to perform the activities or procedures discussed. Such local determinations should be made only with the aid of legal council.

Note: The patients depicted in Case Studies are fictitious.

Library of Congress Cataloging-in-Publication Data

Rahm, Stephen J.
   Pediatric case studies for the paramedic / Stephen J. Rahm. — 1st ed.
      p. ; cm.
   ISBN-13: 978-0-7637-2582-2 (pbk.)   ISBN-10: 0-7637-2582-X (pbk.)
   1. Pediatric emergencies—Case studies. 2. Pediatric emergencies—Problems, exercises, etc. 3. Emergency medical technicians—Case studies. 4. Emergency medical technicians—Problems, exercises, etc.
   I. Title.
   [DNLM: 1. Emergency Treatment—methods—Child—Case Reports.
2. Emergency Treatment—methods—Child—Problems and Exercises.
3. Emergency Treatment—methods—Child, Preschool—Case Reports.
4. Emergency Treatment—methods—Child, Preschool—Problems and Exercises. 5. Emergency Medical Technicians—education—Case Reports.
6. Emergency Medical Technicians—education—Problems and Exercises.
WB 18.2 R147m 2006]
RJ370.R34 2006
618.92'0025—dc22

                                        2005032609   6048

Printed in the United States of America
10 09 08 07 06   10 9 8 7 6 5 4 3 2 1

This book is dedicated to my beautiful children—Eryk, Hailey, and Stephanie. They are the sunshine of my life; I smile every time I think about them and I am proud to be their Dad. I also wish to acknowledge the other important children in my life: my niece, Regan and my nephews—Ryan, Matthew, Casey, and J.T.

CONTENTS

CHAPTER PREVIEW

Pediatric Case Studies for the Paramedic contains 20 case studies representing a variety of pediatric emergencies. Each case study follows a logical and systematic approach to patient assessment and management. Paramedic students apply knowledge from initial training to real-life scenarios as they complete the case studies and answer corresponding questions.

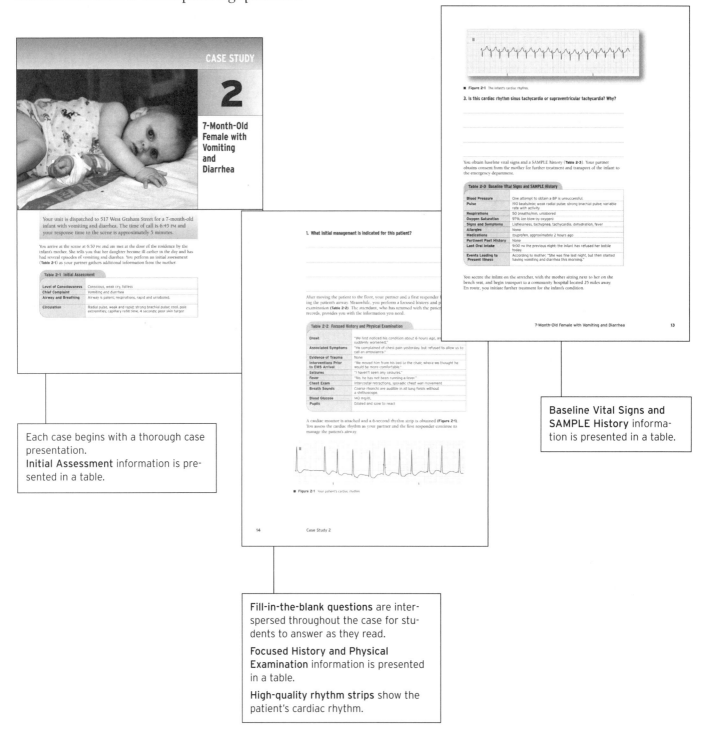

Each case begins with a thorough case presentation.
Initial Assessment information is presented in a table.

Baseline Vital Signs and SAMPLE History information is presented in a table.

Fill-in-the-blank questions are interspersed throughout the case for students to answer as they read.

Focused History and Physical Examination information is presented in a table.

High-quality rhythm strips show the patient's cardiac rhythm.

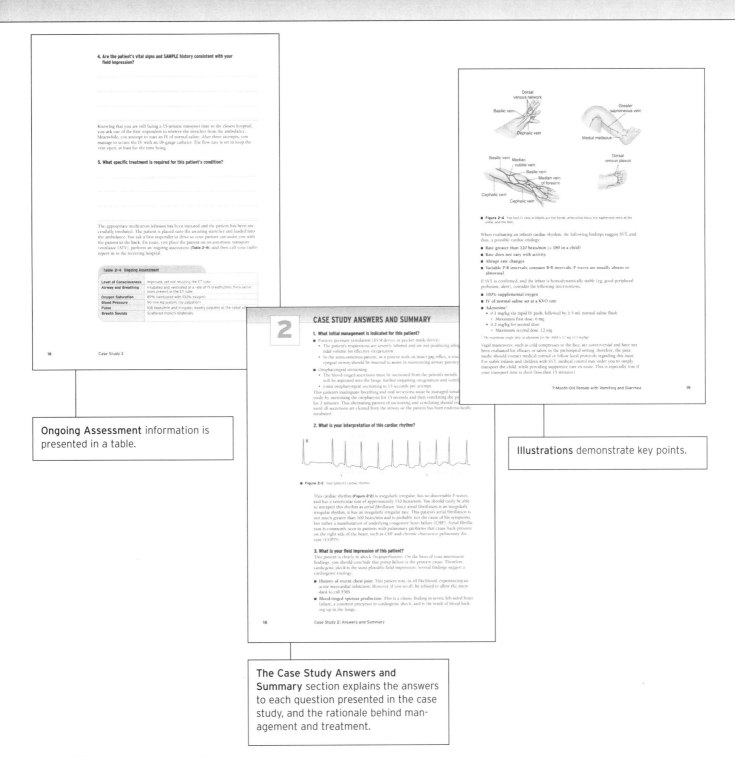

4. Are the patient's vital signs and SAMPLE history consistent with your field impression?

_____

_____

_____

Knowing that you are still facing a 15-minute transport time to the closest hospital, you ask one of the first responders to retrieve the stretcher from the ambulance. Meanwhile, you attempt to start an IV of normal saline. After three attempts, you manage to secure the IV with an 18-gauge catheter. The flow rate is set to keep the vein open, at least for the time being.

5. What specific treatment is required for this patient's condition?

_____

_____

_____

The appropriate medication infusion has been initiated and the patient has been successfully intubated. The patient is placed onto the awaiting stretcher and loaded into the ambulance. You ask a first responder to drive so your partner can assist you with the patient in the back. En route, you place the patient on an automatic transport ventilator (ATV), perform an ongoing assessment **(Table 2-4)**, and then call your radio report in to the receiving hospital.

Table 2-4 Ongoing Assessment

Level of Consciousness	Improved, yet not resisting the ET tube
Airway and Breathing	Intubated and ventilated at a rate of 15 breaths/min; thick secretions present in the ET tube
Oxygen Saturation	89% (ventilated with 100% oxygen)
Blood Pressure	90 mm Hg systolic (by palpation)
Pulse	108 beats/min and irregular; weakly palpable at the radial site
Breath Sounds	Scattered rhonchi bilaterally

16   Case Study 2

Ongoing Assessment information is presented in a table.

Dorsal
venous network

Basilic vein

Cephalic vein

Greater
saphenous vein

Medial malleolus

Basilic vein   Median
cubital vein

Basilic vein

Median vein
of forearm

Cephalic vein

Dorsal
venous plexus

Cephalic vein

■ **Figure 2-4** The best IV sites in infants are the hands, antecubital fossa, the saphenous veins at the ankle, and the feet.

When evaluating an infant's cardiac rhythm, the following findings suggest SVT, and thus, a possible cardiac etiology:

■ Rate greater than 220 beats/min (> 180 in a child)
■ Rate does not vary with activity
■ Abrupt rate changes
■ Variable P-R intervals; constant R-R intervals; P waves are usually absent or abnormal.

If SVT is confirmed, and the infant is hemodynamically stable (eg, good peripheral perfusion, alert), consider the following interventions:

■ 100% supplemental oxygen
■ IV of normal saline set at a KVO rate
■ Adenosine[1]
  • 0.1 mg/kg via rapid IV push, followed by ≥ 5 mL normal saline flush
    • Maximum first dose: 6 mg
  • 0.2 mg/kg for second dose
    • Maximum second dose: 12 mg

[1] The maximum single dose of adenosine for the child is 12 mg (0.3 mg/kg).

Vagal maneuvers, such as cold compresses to the face, are controversial and have not been evaluated for efficacy or safety in the prehospital setting; therefore, the paramedic should contact medical control or follow local protocols regarding this issue. For stable infants and children with SVT, medical control may order you to simply transport the child, while providing supportive care en route. This is especially true if your transport time is short (less than 15 minutes).

7-Month-Old Female with Vomiting and Diarrhea   19

Illustrations demonstrate key points.

2

CASE STUDY ANSWERS AND SUMMARY

1. What initial management is indicated for this patient?

■ Positive pressure ventilation (BVM device or pocket mask device)
  • The patient's respirations are severely labored and are not producing adequate tidal volume for effective oxygenation.
  • In the semiconscious patient, or a patient with an intact gag reflex, a nasopharyngeal airway should be inserted to assist in maintaining airway patency.
■ Oropharyngeal suctioning
  • The blood-tinged secretions must be suctioned from the patient's mouth, will be aspirated into the lungs, further impairing oxygenation and ventilation.
  • Limit oropharyngeal suctioning to 15 seconds per attempt.

This patient's inadequate breathing and oral secretions must be managed simultaneously by suctioning the oropharynx for 15 seconds and then ventilating the patient for 2 minutes. This alternating pattern of suctioning and ventilating should continue until all secretions are cleared from the airway or the patient has been endotracheally intubated.

2. What is your interpretation of this cardiac rhythm?

■ **Figure 2-2** Your patient's cardiac rhythm.

This cardiac rhythm **(Figure 2-2)** is irregularly irregular, has no discernable P waves, and has a ventricular rate of approximately 110 beats/min. You should easily be able to interpret this rhythm as _atrial fibrillation_. Since atrial fibrillation is an irregularly irregular rhythm, it has an irregularly irregular rate. This patient's atrial fibrillation is not much greater than 100 beats/min and is probably not the cause of his symptoms, but rather a manifestation of underlying congestive heart failure (CHF). Atrial fibrillation is commonly seen in patients with pulmonary problems that cause back pressure on the right side of the heart, such as CHF and chronic obstructive pulmonary disease (COPD).

3. What is your field impression of this patient?

This patient is clearly in shock (hypoperfusion). On the basis of your assessment findings, you should conclude that pump failure is the primary cause. Therefore, _cardiogenic shock_ is the most plausible field impression. Several findings suggest a cardiogenic etiology:

■ **History of recent chest pain:** This patient was, in all likelihood, experiencing an acute myocardial infarction. However, if you recall, he refused to allow the attendant to call EMS.
■ **Blood-tinged sputum production:** This is a classic finding in severe left-sided heart failure, a common precursor to cardiogenic shock, and is the result of blood backing up in the lungs.

18   Case Study 2: Answers and Summary

The **Case Study Answers and Summary** section explains the answers to each question presented in the case study, and the rationale behind management and treatment.

Other titles in the Case Studies series include:

Medical Case Studies for the Paramedic
ISBN: 0-7637-2581-1

Trauma Case Studies for the Paramedic
ISBN: 0-7637-2583-8

ACKNOWLEDGMENTS

Jones and Bartlett Publishers would like to thank the following people for reviewing this text:

Sandra Hartley, MS, CP
Pensacola Junior College
Pensacola, Florida

Mark A. Huckaby, NREMT-P
Grant Medical Center
Columbus, Ohio

Sue Kartman, CCEMT-P
Madison Area Technical College
Madison, Wisconsin

Greg Mullen
National EMS Academy
Lafayette, Louisiana

Manish Shah, MD
Pediatric Emergency Medicine
Texas Children's Hospital
Houston, Texas

Jeffrey J. Spencer
Director of Paramedic Education
LaGuardia Community College/CUNY
Long Island City, New York

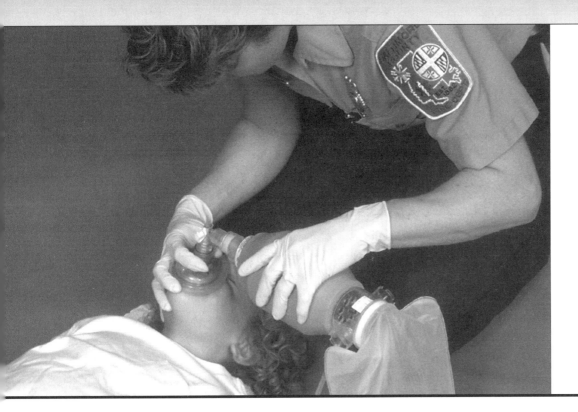

Introduction

Clearly, children are not simply small adults. They commonly present with unique problems that are typically not encountered in older patients. These unique problems require the paramedic to alter, to some degree, his or her approach to the sick or injured child. To facilitate a better understanding of caring for children, programs such as *Pediatric Education for Prehospital Professionals* (PEPP) have been developed.

Because a relatively small percentage of EMS calls involve a critically ill or injured child, it is quite common for the paramedic to experience anxiety when such a call is received. An understanding of the anatomic and physiologic differences between pediatric and adult patients, however, will allow the paramedic to make necessary adjustments in assessment and management strategies, thereby maximizing his or her ability to effectively care for their younger counterparts.

Pediatric Case Studies for the Paramedic contains 20 case studies, representing a variety of pediatric medical and trauma emergencies that the paramedic may encounter in the field.

How to use this book

Pediatric Case Studies for the Paramedic is intended to reinforce to paramedic students the importance of a systematic patient assessment and management approach by presenting them with pediatric medical and trauma emergencies that they are likely to encounter in the field. This book should be used as an additional resource for the paramedic student to test newly gained knowledge and prepare for examinations; it should not be used in place of a primary paramedic textbook.

Each case study will begin by presenting you with dispatch information, just as you would receive on an actual call, and a general impression of the patient upon arriving at the scene. Then, as the case progresses, pertinent patient information will be provided, interspersed with a series of questions designed to test your knowledge of the patient's illness or injury and respective treatment.

A suggested method for using this book is to read each part of the scenario, and then, in the area provided, answer the question that follows in as much detail as possible prior to reading the next part of the case study. Your detailed response to the questions will help reinforce your knowledge of the material. Continue this until you have read all of the scenario information and answered all of the case study questions. You should then compare your answers to those outlined in the case summary that immediately follows each case study.

The case summary provides answers to the questions asked within the case, as well as additional enrichment information, to include the following:

- Additional signs and symptoms commonly associated with the patient's illness or injury
- Information and justification for each treatment modality
- Specific considerations for dealing with the pediatric patient
- Basic pathophysiology of the patient's illness or injury

Treatment Guidelines

The treatment recommendations contained within this book conform to the current standards of care as outlined in the following:

- U.S. DOT EMT-Paramedic National Standard Curriculum, revised 1998
- American Heart Association and American Academy of Pediatrics Guidelines and Algorithms, revised 2005
- Brain Trauma Foundation (BTF), 2004

Additional treatment or variations in treatment may be required for the conditions presented in this book. As with the management of any patient, the paramedic must conform to the protocols inherent to their EMS system, and should contact medical control as needed.

Body Substance Isolation (BSI) Precautions and Scene Safety

Strict adherence to proper body substance isolation (BSI) precautions and constantly observing the scene for safety hazards is of paramount importance when managing any patient. Throughout each of the case studies presented in this book, it is assumed that the proper BSI precautions are being followed at all times. Unless otherwise stated in the case study, it is also assumed that the scene is safe for you to enter.

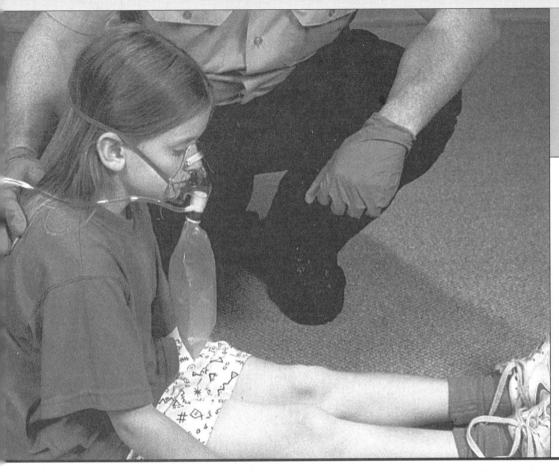

1

7-Year-Old Female with Difficulty Breathing

At 8:45 AM, your unit is dispatched to Fabra Elementary School for a 7-year-old female with difficulty breathing. The outside temperature is 35°F following the recent passage of a cold front. Your response time to the scene is approximately 3 minutes.

Upon arriving at the scene, you are greeted by the school nurse, who tells you that the girl entered her office with mild respiratory distress. The nurse further tells you that the child's temperature was 97.8°F (oral). You introduce yourself to the patient and perform an initial assessment (**Table 1-1**). Your partner begins to initiate treatment.

Table 1-1 Initial Assessment

Level of Consciousness	Conscious and alert to person, place, and time; fearful
Chief Complaint	"I am having trouble breathing and forgot my medicine at home."
Airway and Breathing	Airway patent; respirations, increased and labored; adequate air movement
Circulation	Radial pulse increased, strong, and regular; skin is pink, warm, and dry; no gross bleeding

1. What initial management is indicated for this child?

_____

_____

_____

_____

The patient is tolerant of your initial treatment and remains conscious and alert. She tells you that she has a "breathing problem" and takes medicine for it. However, she cannot recall the name of the medication. As the school nurse attempts to contact the patient's mother, you perform a focused history and physical examination (**Table 1-2**).

Table 1-2 Focused History and Physical Examination

Onset	"This started really fast."
Provocation/Palliation	"I started coughing real bad and then I started having trouble breathing."
Quality	"It feels like I can't get all the air out of my chest."
Severity	"This is not the worst breathing trouble that I have had."
Time	"This started right after I got to school."
Interventions Prior to EMS Arrival	None
Chest Exam	Chest moves symmetrically; slight intercostal retractions; no obvious trauma
Breath Sounds	Audible expiratory wheezing
Oxygen Saturation	91% (on 100% oxygen)

2. What is your field impression of this child?

_____

_____

_____

_____

You proceed to obtain baseline vital signs and a SAMPLE history (**Table 1-3**) as your partner prepares to initiate further treatment. The nurse states that she has contacted the child's mother, who wishes for you to take her to the hospital where she will meet you.

Table 1-3 Baseline Vital Signs and SAMPLE History

Blood Pressure	96/56 mm Hg
Pulse	130 beats/min, strong and regular
Respirations	30 breaths/min, labored
Oxygen Saturation	91% (on 100% oxygen)
Signs and Symptoms	Difficulty breathing, intercostal retractions, low oxygen saturation, wheezing
Allergies	None
Medications	"I take medicine whenever this happens, but I don't know what it is called."
Pertinent Past History	"I have breathing problems like this every once in a while."
Last Oral Intake	"I had a bowl of cereal before I came to school."
Events Leading to Present Illness	"I started coughing really bad, and then I couldn't breathe."

3. Are the child's vital signs and SAMPLE history consistent with your field impression?

The girl, clearly frightened, asks you if you are going to stick her with a needle. You tell her that you don't think that will be necessary. However, you do tell her that you are going to give her a "breathing treatment" that will hopefully make her feel better. You apply a cardiac monitor, which reveals a sinus tachycardia at 130 beats/min.

4. What specific treatment is indicated for this child's condition?

The patient's condition has improved following your intervention. She is no longer retracting and her oxygen saturation has increased to 94%. You reauscultate her lungs and note the presence of scattered expiratory wheezing. After loading the patient into the ambulance, you proceed to a hospital located 15 miles away. En route, you perform an ongoing assessment (**Table 1-4**).

Table 1-4 Ongoing Assessment

Level of Consciousness	Conscious and alert to person, place, and time; calm
Airway and Breathing	Airway remains patent; respirations, 24 breaths/min; unlabored
Oxygen Saturation	94% (on 100% oxygen)
Blood Pressure	90 mm Hg systolic (by palpation)
Pulse	130 beats/min, strong and regular
Breath Sounds	Scattered expiratory wheezing (bilaterally)
ECG	Sinus tachycardia

5. Is additional treatment required for this child?

_____

_____

_____

The patient's condition continues to improve en route to the hospital. Her oxygen saturation is 98% and her breath sounds are clear to auscultation bilaterally. You call your radio report to the receiving facility and give them an estimated time of arrival of 5 minutes.

6. Are there any special considerations for this child?

_____

_____

_____

The child is delivered to the emergency department in stable condition. You give your verbal report to the attending physician, who has already gathered the child's medical history from her mother. Following additional treatment in the emergency department, the child is discharged home.

1. What initial management is indicated for this child?

- **100% supplemental oxygen (via pediatric nonrebreathing mask)**
  - Though clearly experiencing respiratory distress, this patient's respiratory effort is producing adequate air movement. Therefore, positive-pressure ventilation support is not needed at this time.

You must carefully monitor the child with respiratory distress and be prepared to provide positive-pressure ventilations if signs of respiratory failure develop. Signs of respiratory failure include, among others, reduced tidal volume and poor air movement, decreased level of consciousness, a low (> 90%) or rapidly falling oxygen saturation, and signs of physical exhaustion.

Failure of the respiratory system is the most common cause of cardiac arrest in the pediatric population. However, with frequent respiratory system assessments and prompt management, this potential catastrophe can often be prevented.

2. What is your field impression of this child?

You should suspect that this child is experiencing an acute asthma attack. In addition to the complaint of difficulty breathing, the following pertinent findings support this field impression:

- **Expiratory wheezing,** which is a hallmark sign of a mild to moderate asthma attack. Expiratory wheezing indicates impaired airflow during expiration and is indicative of bronchospasm.
  - By no means is wheezing exclusive to asthma. Other conditions, such as pneumonia and toxic inhalations, cause wheezing as well. However, the clinical scenario involving this patient does not indicate a toxic exposure and the fact that she is afebrile (97.8°F) is not consistent with pneumonia or other infectious causes of respiratory distress.
- **Cold air exposure,** which is a common precipitant to an asthma attack. Like any other smooth muscle, the smooth muscle surrounding the bronchiole constricts when exposed to cold air.
- **Prescribed medications,** which indicate the presence of an episodic disease that requires periodic treatment. Other respiratory illnesses, such as croup, bronchitis, and pneumonia, are typically treated with a trial of medications, and usually resolve without the need for ongoing treatment.
- **The nature of onset,** which, in this patient, was coughing. As the bronchioles become irritated, the patient often begins to cough, sometimes violently. Then, as bronchospasm progresses, respiratory distress develops.

Asthma is the most common chronic childhood disease, affecting approximately 5 million American children over 1 year of age. Nearly half of all pediatric asthma deaths occur in the prehospital setting.

Asthma is a chronic but reversible condition, characterized by bronchospasm, mucous plugging, and edema in the lower airways (**Figure 1-1**). Asthma is commonly referred to as reactive airway disease (RAD)—a nonspecific condition in which intrinsic or extrinsic factors cause bronchospasm—at least initially, until a physician determines that the patient has met all of the diagnostic criteria for asthma.

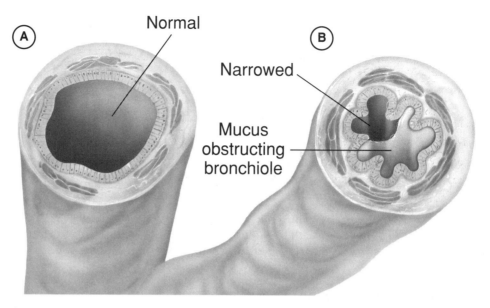

Normal

A Narrowed B

Mucus obstructing bronchiole

■ **Figure 1-1** Asthma is an acute spasm of the bronchioles. (A) Cross-section of a normal bronchiole. (B) The bronchiole in spasm; a mucous plug has formed and partially obstructed the bronchiole.

An acute asthma attack is commonly precipitated by factors such as an allergen exposure, stress, exercise, recent upper respiratory infections, and exposure to cold air or passive cigarette smoke. In response to the precipitating event, a series of reactions occur in the lower airway. First, the smooth muscle surrounding the bronchiole begins to spasm, resulting in bronchoconstriction. Secondly, mucous glands and cells that line the lower airway secrete excessive mucous, which accumulates in the bronchioles, creating a plug. Finally, fluid shifts into the walls of the lower airway, resulting in edema that further decreases the diameter of the bronchiole. The net result is a narrowing of the small airways with increased resistance to airflow.

These three factors—bronchospasm, mucous plugging, and airway edema—result in a ventilation-perfusion mismatch. In other words, the pathophysiologic changes associated with asthma cause some alveoli to become hyperinflated due to air trapping, while other alveoli collapse (atelectasis). Hypoxemia develops because the collapsed alveoli are still being perfused, but are unable to participate in gas exchange. Therefore, the blood flowing through the capillaries adjacent to the collapsed alveoli returns to the left side of the heart, still unoxygenated. This condition is referred to as intrapulmonary shunting.

In between attacks, the child with asthma is typically asymptomatic. However, during an acute attack, varying degrees of difficulty breathing, tachypnea, tachycardia, and wheezing are present.

As a baseline, an acute asthma attack presents with some degree of respiratory distress. The presence of wheezing often characterizes the severity of the attack, and thus, the degree of bronchoconstriction. In a mild to moderate asthma attack, wheezing is typically audible at the end of expiration, indicating increased resistance to expiratory airflow. Oxygen saturation levels may be normal (≥ 95%) or slightly low.

During a more severe asthma attack, wheezing may be audible during inspiration and expiration. Oxygen saturation levels typically reflect mild hypoxemia, with readings that usually range from 91% to 94%.

Status asthmaticus, the most severe exacerbation of asthma, is a life-threatening condition that often requires multiple modalities of frequent or continuous treatment to improve. The child with status asthmaticus presents with air hunger (struggling to breathe). However, because of the profound bronchoconstriction and minimal airflow through the bronchioles, wheezing is either faint or completely absent. Oxygen saturation levels often reflect severe hypoxia, with readings well below 90%. As hypoxemia worsens, hypercarbia (increased arterial CO_2 levels) develops and the child may become unresponsive.

Table 1-5 lists the common clinical findings associated with asthma. Bear in mind, however, that the severity of the attack will determine which clinical findings are present.

Table 1-5 Clinical Findings Associated with Asthma

Respiratory distress
Intercostal retractions
Nasal flaring
Tachypnea • Bradypnea is an ominous sign and indicates impending respiratory arrest.
Episodes of coughing
Wheezing • Expiratory during a mild to moderate attack • Inspiratory and expiratory during a more severe attack • Faint or absent during status asthmaticus
Tachycardia • Bradycardia in the child is almost always the result of profound hypoxia and indicates impending respiratory or cardiac arrest.
Cyanosis (late sign)
Fluctuations in oxygen saturation • Normal or slightly low during mild attacks • 91% to 94% during moderate attacks • Less than 90% during severe attacks

3. Are the child's vital signs and SAMPLE history consistent with your field impression?

According to the following formula, this child's blood pressure of 96/56 mm Hg is consistent with her age:

$$\text{Age [in years]} \times 2 + 70 = \text{systolic blood pressure}$$

Her heart rate and respiratory rate, however, indicate respiratory distress. Additionally, her oxygen saturation of 93% indicates mild hypoxemia.

Although she cannot remember the name of her medication, the fact that she has prescribed medications is an indicator of an episodic disease that requires periodic treatment, such as asthma. Additionally, she has confirmed that her doctor told her that she has a "breathing problem."

As previously discussed, her episode of coughing prior to developing respiratory distress is a fairly common finding in patients with asthma.

4. What specific treatment is indicated for this child's condition?

The goals of asthma treatment are to relieve bronchospasm and hypoxemia and to improve ventilation. In addition to supplemental oxygen, this is most effectively accomplished, at least initially, with a selective beta$_2$ agonist.

Albuterol (Proventil, Ventolin) is the most popular inhaled bronchodilator because of its selective action on the bronchiole smooth muscle. Albuterol is administered via nebulizer in a concentration of 5 mg/mL (0.5%) or via metered dose inhaler (MDI) in a concentration of 90 μg per puff. Pediatric doses for albuterol are as follows:

- Nebulizer
  - < 15 kg (< 33 lbs): 2.5–5 mg (0.5–1 mL) diluted in 3 mL of normal saline, nebulized; repeated every 20 minutes up to three doses
    - Administer continuously in critical patients.
  - > 15 kg (> 33 lbs): 5–10 mg (1–2 mL) diluted in 3 mL of normal saline, nebulized; repeated every 20 minutes up to three doses
    - Administer continuously in critical patients.
- MDI (all weights and ages)
  - 4–8 puffs every 20 minutes up to three doses; administer with a mask or spacer device (**Figure 1-2**)

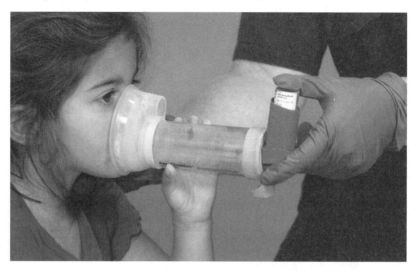

■ **Figure 1-2** A metered dose inhaler and spacer device can be used with or without a mask.

Other selective beta$_2$ agonists, such as metaproterenol (Alupent), isoetharine (Bronkosol), and terbutaline (Brethine), are also used in the treatment of asthma. Ipratropium bromide (Atrovent), an anticholinergic bronchodilator, is an adjunct medication used in the treatment of asthma. Refer to locally established protocols regarding the pediatric doses of these drugs.

If a child cannot tolerate inhaled bronchodilator therapy, or is moving air so poorly that the drug is not being effectively inhaled, epinephrine 1:1,000 (1 mg/mL) should be administered in the following dose:

- **0.01 mg/kg via SQ injection, repeated every 20 minutes up to three doses**
  - Maximum single dose of 0.3 mg (0.3 mL)

Corticosteroids, such as methylprednisolone (Solu-Medrol), should be used in conjunction with beta$_2$ agonists for moderate to severe asthma attacks. Follow locally established protocols regarding administration of steroids in the treatment of asthma.

Agitation in the child can increase oxygen demand and consumption, potentially resulting in deterioration of his or her condition. For this reason, painful procedures, such as IV therapy, should be reserved for critically ill children that may require IV-administered medications. If IV therapy is indicated, use normal saline and the appropriate-sized pediatric catheter. If IV access is not possible in the critically ill child, an intraosseous cannula should be inserted.

A cardiac monitor should be placed on any patient with respiratory distress, pediatric or otherwise. Although ventricular arrhythmias (eg, V-fib, V-tach) are highly uncommon in children, the cardiac monitor serves as an excellent means of monitoring the child's heart rate, especially for bradycardia, which would indicate impending respiratory or cardiac arrest.

5. Is additional treatment required for this child?

Your patient's condition has clearly improved following the first bronchodilator treatment; however, you are still 15 miles away from the hospital and, as evidenced by the scattered wheezing and oxygen saturation of 94%, her attack has not completely resolved. In addition to continuing oxygen therapy, at least one more bronchodilator treatment is indicated, with the goals being to resolve the wheezing and maintain her oxygen saturation level at 95% or higher.

6. Are there any special considerations for this child?

Because of the severe air trapping associated with bronchospasm, positive-pressure ventilation is associated with potential complications in the asthma patient. Positive-pressure ventilation requires very high inspiratory pressures and may result in pneumothorax or pneumomediastinum through a process called the "paper bag" effect. In other words, the hyperinflated alveoli can rupture when exposed to high inspiratory airway pressures, causing air to enter the pleural space or mediastinum. Consider bag-valve-mask ventilation of an asthmatic child only if the child is in respiratory failure and has failed to respond to maximal bronchodilator therapy.

You must always be prepared for the child to develop status asthmaticus, even if he or she appears to be responding favorably to therapy. In the focused exam, the following historical findings should increase your index of suspicion for this potentially lethal event:

- Prior ICU admissions or intubation
- More than three emergency department visits in the past year
- More than two hospital admissions in the past year
- Use of more than one metered-dose inhaler canister in the last month
- Use of steroids for asthma in the past
- Use of bronchodilators more frequently than every 4 hours
- Progressive symptoms despite aggressive home therapy

Summary

Asthma, a reactive disease of the lower airways, is the most common chronic disease of childhood. Asthma is characterized by bronchospasm, mucous plugging, and airway edema. An asthma attack is commonly precipitated by events such as stress, exercise, recent upper respiratory infection, and exposure to cold air or passive cigarette smoke.

The clinical presentation of asthma depends on the severity of bronchospasm and bronchiole inflammation. Clinical presentations range from a child who is mildly dyspneic with scattered expiratory wheezing to one who is struggling to breathe, has faint or absent wheezing, and a decreased level of consciousness secondary to severe hypoxia and acidosis.

Initial treatment for asthma includes ensuring airway patency and administering 100% supplemental oxygen. If signs of respiratory failure are present, positive-pressure ventilation may be needed. Initial pharmacological management typically involves the administration of a selective beta$_2$ agonist, such as albuterol, Alupent, or Bronkosol, administered via nebulizer or MDI.

Other pharmacological management may include corticosteroids (ie, Solu-Medrol), anticholinergic bronchodilators (ie, Atrovent), or other beta$_2$ agonists (ie, Brethine), especially if the child's condition is refractory to other treatment and/or your transport time to the hospital will be prolonged. Refer to locally established protocols or contact medical control as needed regarding additional treatment for pediatric asthma.

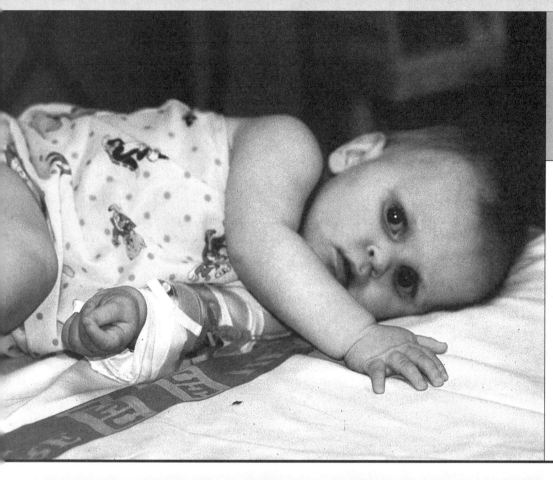

2

7-Month-Old Female with Vomiting and Diarrhea

Your unit is dispatched to 517 West Graham Street for a 7-month-old infant with vomiting and diarrhea. The time of call is 6:45 PM and your response time to the scene is approximately 5 minutes.

You arrive at the scene at 6:50 PM and are met at the door of the residence by the infant's mother. She tells you that her daughter became ill earlier in the day and has had several episodes of vomiting and diarrhea. You perform an initial assessment (Table 2-1) as your partner gathers additional information from the mother.

Table 2-1 Initial Assessment

Level of Consciousness	Conscious, weak cry, listless
Chief Complaint	Vomiting and diarrhea
Airway and Breathing	Airway is patent; respirations, rapid and unlabored.
Circulation	Radial pulse, weak and rapid; strong brachial pulse; cool, pale extremities; capillary refill time, 4 seconds; poor skin turgor

1. What initial management is indicated for this infant?

_____

_____

_____

_____

With the assistance of the mother, your partner has begun the appropriate initial management. The mother tells you that her daughter has been running a fever of 101.5°F, which she treated with ibuprofen. She further tells you that she has attempted to give the infant Pedialyte and water; however, the infant has refused to take her bottle. You perform a focused history and physical examination (**Table 2-2**) with information gathered from the mother.

Table 2-2 Focused History and Physical Examination

Onset	"This started quite suddenly. She was fine last night."
Time	"This started about 6:30 this morning."
Severity	"She vomited three times and has had at least five episodes of diarrhea."
Associated Symptoms	Rectal temperature, 101.5°F
Blood Glucose	90 mg/dL
Abdominal Exam	Abdomen is soft; the infant does not cry when her abdomen is palpated.

2. What is your initial impression of this infant?

_____

_____

_____

_____

Because of the infant's rapid heart rate, you apply a cardiac monitor and assess her cardiac rhythm (**Figure 2-1**). The infant's mother asks if you suspect a heart problem, but you assure her that you are merely evaluating her daughter's heart rate. You note variation in the rate of the infant's cardiac rhythm when she moves.

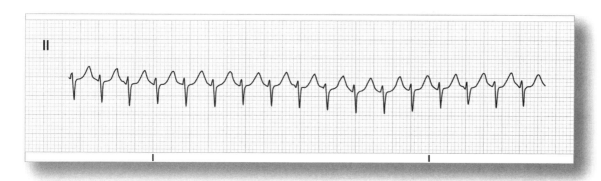

■ **Figure 2-1** The infant's cardiac rhythm.

3. Is this cardiac rhythm sinus tachycardia or supraventricular tachycardia? Why?

_____

_____

_____

_____

You obtain baseline vital signs and a SAMPLE history (**Table 2-3**). Your partner obtains consent from the mother for further treatment and transport of the infant to the emergency department.

Table 2-3 Baseline Vital Signs and SAMPLE History

Blood Pressure	One attempt to obtain a BP is unsuccessful.
Pulse	190 beats/min; weak radial pulse; strong brachial pulse; variable rate with activity
Respirations	50 breaths/min, unlabored
Oxygen Saturation	97% (on blow-by oxygen)
Signs and Symptoms	Listlessness, tachypnea, tachycardia, dehydration, fever
Allergies	None
Medications	Ibuprofen, approximately 2 hours ago
Pertinent Past History	None
Last Oral Intake	9:00 PM the previous night; the infant has refused her bottle today.
Events Leading to Present Illness	According to mother, "She was fine last night, but then started having vomiting and diarrhea this morning."

You secure the infant on the stretcher, with the mother sitting next to her on the bench seat, and begin transport to a community hospital located 25 miles away. En route, you initiate further treatment for the infant's condition.

4. What specific treatment is indicated for this infant?

_____

_____

_____

_____

The infant's condition improves with your treatment interventions. Her extremities are not as pale and her capillary refill time is 2 to 3 seconds. Following additional treatment, you perform an ongoing assessment (**Table 2-4**) and then call your radio report to the receiving facility. Your estimated time of arrival is 10 minutes.

Table 2-4 Ongoing Assessment

Level of Consciousness	Conscious, increased activity
Airway and Breathing	Airway remains patent; respirations, 40 breaths/min and unlabored
Oxygen Saturation	98% (on blow-by oxygen)
Pulse	140 beats/min, strong and regular
ECG	Normal sinus rhythm
Blood Glucose	98 mg/dL

You deliver the infant to the emergency department and give your verbal report to the charge nurse. The infant was diagnosed with viral gastroenteritis and given additional treatment in the emergency department. She was admitted for fluid and electrolyte replenishment and later discharged home.

5. How would your management have differed if this infant's tachycardia was cardiac-related?

_____

_____

_____

_____

2

1. What initial management is indicated for this infant?

- 100% supplemental oxygen (pediatric nonrebreathing mask or blow-by technique)
  - Effortless (without difficulty) tachypnea is a sign of decreased perfusion, and should be treated with supplemental oxygen.

At present, this infant's respirations, though increased, are unlabored. Therefore, positive-pressure ventilatory support is not required at this time. You must closely monitor this infant for signs of respiratory failure, and be prepared to support ventilations. Signs of respiratory failure in infants and children include the following:

- Decreased alertness
- Signs of exhaustion
- Cyanosis
- Bradycardia
- Reduced tidal volume (shallow breathing)

Applying oxygen to infants and young children may cause agitation, thus increasing oxygen demand and consumption. In the already hypoperfused child, this could result in deterioration of his or her condition. You must therefore administer oxygen in a manner that is nonthreatening.

If a child resists the use of an oxygen mask, have the parent give blow-by oxygen from the end of the oxygen tubing or from tubing inserted into a cup. This method of oxygen delivery is beneficial in two ways—it is usually well tolerated by the child, and it helps to alleviate parent anxiety by allowing them to participate in the care of their child.

2. What is your initial impression of this infant?

This infant is *severely dehydrated* and is experiencing signs of *early (compensated) shock*. The following clinical findings support this field impression:

- Listlessness
- Tachypnea
- Tachycardia
- Weak peripheral (radial) pulse; strong central (brachial) pulse
- Cool, pale extremities
- Delayed capillary refill

Compensated shock (hypoperfusion) occurs when there is inadequate perfusion of the body's tissues; however, the body is able to maintain core perfusion by shunting blood from the periphery to the vital organs. In the infant or small child, compensated shock indicates the loss of approximately 15% of their circulating volume. The signs of compensated shock (**Table 2-5**) indicate decreased cerebral perfusion and the release of catecholamines (epinephrine and norepinephrine) from the sympathetic nervous system, which increases the heart rate and "clamps down" the peripheral vasculature.

Table 2-5 Signs of Compensated Shock

Irritability
Tachypnea
Tachycardia
Weak peripheral pulses, but strong central pulses
Delayed (> 2 seconds) capillary refill
Cool, pale extremities
Decreased urine output
Normal systolic blood pressure

Because blood pressure is often difficult to obtain in children under 3 years of age, you should focus your assessment on other indicators of perfusion. These include pulse strength, capillary refill time, and level of alertness. Hypotension, which indicates decompensated shock, represents the loss of at least 25% of the pediatric patient's circulating volume.

Viral gastroenteritis is the most common cause of dehydration and hypovolemic shock in infants and small children. During gastroenteritis, microorganisms invade the gastrointestinal tract, where they release toxic substances that irritate the gastric and intestinal linings. This causes an immediate loss of water and electrolytes from the body through vomiting and diarrhea. Fever, which is often present with viral gastroenteritis, causes further loss of water from the body.

Dehydration is classified as being mild, moderate, and severe, with the clinical presentation indicating the severity of dehydration. In addition to the signs of shock, severe dehydration in the infant is characterized by dry mucous membranes, sunken eyes, furrowed tongue, sunken anterior fontanel, and poor skin turgor (**Figure 2-2**).

Infants and children are at greater risk than adults for dehydration because their fluid reserves are smaller and rapidly depleted. Relative to adults, infants and children can succumb to severe dehydration within a matter of hours.

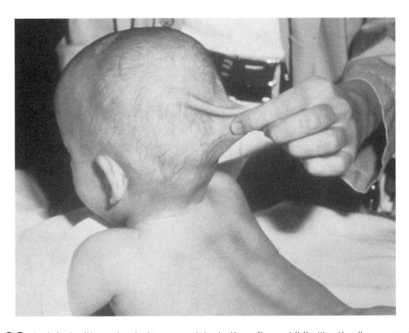

■ **Figure 2-2** An infant with moderate to severe dehydration often exhibits "tenting," or poor skin turgor. This indicates decreased skin elasticity secondary to fluid loss.

3. Is this cardiac rhythm sinus tachycardia or supraventricular tachycardia? Why?

The rhythm depicted in **Figure 2-3** is sinus tachycardia at a rate of approximately 195 beats/min. Sinus tachycardia is not an arrhythmia per se; it is a response to an underlying etiology. In this infant, the tachycardia is a compensatory response to a combination of severe dehydration, hypovolemia, and fever. Other causes of sinus tachycardia include fear, pain, and hypoxia.

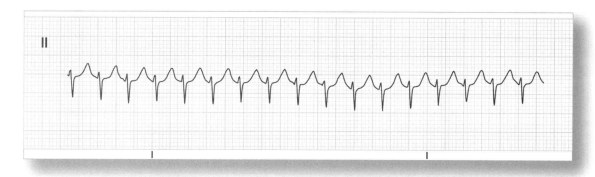

■ **Figure 2-3** Sinus tachycardia.

Most tachycardias in children are sinus tachycardia; however, you should still consider evaluating the cardiac rhythm in any child that presents with tachycardia. Although highly doubtful in this case, some tachycardias in children are supraventricular in origin, and thus, suggest a cardiac etiology.

Unlike supraventricular tachycardia (SVT), the rate of sinus tachycardia varies with activity, which is evidenced by a varying R-R interval. P waves are usually present and of consistent shape and the P-R intervals are consistent in length. Additionally, the tachycardia typically begins to resolve once treatment of the underlying problem is initiated (eg, IV fluids, oxygen, antipyretics).

In infants, tachycardia that is less than 220 beats/min, especially in the presence of fever, pain, hypovolemia, or hypoxia, is almost always sinus tachycardia. **Table 2-6** provides a differential diagnosis of tachycardia in the infant.

Table 2-6 Distinguishing Pediatric Sinus Tachycardia from Supraventricular Tachycardia

Sinus Tachycardia
- Compatible or suggestive history:
  - Fever
  - Pain
  - Hypoxia
  - Volume loss
- Heart rate is less than 220 beats/min in infants; less than 180 beats/min in children.
- Heart rate varies with activity.
- Varying R-R intervals, constant P-R intervals, P waves present
- Assessment findings
  - Hypovolemia
  - Hypoxia
  - Painful injury
  - Hemodynamic compromise
    - Caused by the underlying problem (eg, shock, hypoxia) rather than the tachycardia itself

(Continued)

Table 2-6 Distinguishing Pediatric Sinus Tachycardia from Supraventricular Tachycardia (Continued)

Supraventricular Tachycardia (SVT)
- Incompatible history for sinus tachycardia:
  - Congenital heart disease
  - Known SVT
  - Nonspecific symptoms (eg, poor feeding, fussiness)
- Heart rate is greater than 220 beats/min in infants; greater than 180 beats/min in children.
  - Can be as high as 240–300 beats/min in infants
- Heart rate does not vary with activity.
- Abrupt heart rate changes (paroxysms)
- Constant R-R intervals; varying P-R intervals; P waves are usually absent or abnormal.
- Assessment findings
  - CHF may be present.
  - Hemodynamic compromise
    - Caused by the tachycardia itself

4. What specific treatment is indicated for this infant?

Due to the severe dehydration and signs of compensated shock, as well as your extended transport time (25 miles), IV fluid replacement is indicated for this infant. As recommended by the American Academy of Pediatrics (AAP), you should initiate IV therapy en route to the hospital in infants and children who are in compensated shock.

IV therapy in the infant or small child can clearly be time-consuming and can result in unnecessary delays at the scene. During this time, the infant could develop decompensated shock, resulting in venous collapse that would only hamper your efforts to locate a suitable vein.

Isotonic crystalloid solutions, such as normal saline or lactated Ringer's solution, are the preferred fluids to use for volume replacement. In the infant or child, infuse 20 mL/kg over 10–20 minutes and then reassess. Give additional fluid boluses as needed if the infant does not respond.

The best IV sites in infants are the hands, antecubital fossa, saphenous vein at the ankle, and feet (**Figure 2-4**). If peripheral IV access is unsuccessful after 3 attempts or 90 seconds, insert an intraosseous catheter.

Although fluid overload in a severely dehydrated infant with shock is unlikely with 2 or 3 boluses of IV crystalloid, using a special type of microdrip set called a volutrol (buretrol) allows you to fill the large drip chamber with a specific amount of fluid and administer only that amount to avoid fluid overload. The 100-mL calibrated drip chamber can be shut off from the IV bag. The large drip chamber can be refilled as needed for additional fluid boluses.

An additional protective measure to assess for early signs of fluid overload would be to auscultate the infant or child's lungs, especially following 3 or 4 fluid boluses.

5. How would your management have differed if this infant's tachycardia was cardiac-related?

As previously discussed, tachycardia in infants and children is almost always sinus tachycardia and is a compensatory response to an underlying problem (eg, shock, hypoxia, fever). However, in the absence of any underlying problems that would explain the tachycardia, you should perform a careful, systematic assessment to detect signs of hemodynamic instability related to the tachycardia. During the focused exam, inquire about a history of congenital heart problems or SVT.

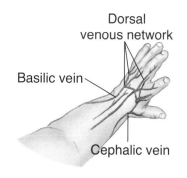
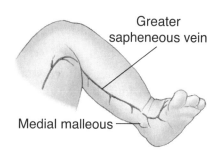
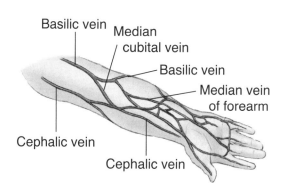
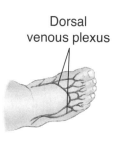

■ **Figure 2-4** The best IV sites in infants are the hands, antecubital fossa, the saphenous veins at the ankle, and the feet.

When evaluating an infant's cardiac rhythm, the following findings suggest SVT, and thus, a possible cardiac etiology:

■ Rate greater than 220 beats/min (> 180 in a child)

■ Rate does not vary with activity.

■ Abrupt rate changes

■ Variable P-R intervals; constant R-R intervals; P waves are usually absent or abnormal.

If SVT is confirmed, and the infant is hemodynamically stable (eg, good peripheral perfusion, alert), consider the following interventions:

■ 100% supplemental oxygen

■ IV of normal saline set at a KVO rate

■ Adenosine
  • 0.1 mg/kg via rapid IV push, followed by ≥ 5 mL normal saline flush
    • Maximum first dose: 6 mg
  • 0.2 mg/kg for second dose
    • Maximum second dose: 12 mg

Vagal maneuvers, such as cold compresses to the face, are controversial and have not been evaluated for efficacy or safety in the prehospital setting; therefore, the paramedic should contact medical control or follow local protocols regarding this issue. For stable infants and children with SVT, medical control may order you to simply transport the child, while providing supportive care en route. This is especially true if your transport time is short (less than 15 minutes).

If an infant or child with SVT is hemodynamically unstable (eg, unconscious, poor perfusion), the following interventions should be performed:

- **100% supplemental oxygen**
  - Support ventilations if the child is breathing inadequately
- **IV/IO of normal saline set at a KVO rate**
- **Synchronized cardioversion**[1]
  - 0.5–1 joule/kg
    - Repeat at 2 joules/kg if needed.

[1] *Consider adenosine prior to performing cardioversion **only** if IV/IO access is already obtained. DO NOT delay cardioversion for the purpose of establishing vascular access.*

Summary

In the absence of trauma, shock in the pediatric population is almost always the result of dehydration caused by severe vomiting, diarrhea, or both. Viral gastroenteritis is a common mechanism for fluid loss in pediatric patients.

In the infant, signs of significant dehydration include dry mucous membranes, poor skin turgor, sunken eyes and anterior fontanel, and decreased urine output.

Because of their relatively small fluid reserves, shock will develop much faster in infants and children than in adults. During early (compensated) shock, the infant or child will present with signs of decreased peripheral perfusion, such as tachycardia with weak peripheral pulses (strong central pulses), pale and cool extremities, and delayed capillary refill. These signs indicate the shunting of peripheral blood flow to the core of the body, where the vital organs are located.

Unless promptly treated, decompensated shock will develop quickly in infants and children, resulting in cardiovascular collapse and death. Signs of decompensated shock include a decreased level of consciousness, tachycardia with weak central pulses, profoundly delayed capillary refill, and hypotension.

Following assessment of airway, breathing, and circulation, and the correction of immediate life-threatening problems, treatment for pediatric dehydration and shock includes supplemental oxygen and IV crystalloid boluses of 20 mL/kg. Consider the use of a Volutrol microdrip set to prevent inadvertent fluid overload; frequent assessment of breath sounds is also advisable. Transport the child to the closest appropriate facility for continued fluid rehydration, electrolyte stabilization, and treatment of his or her underlying condition.

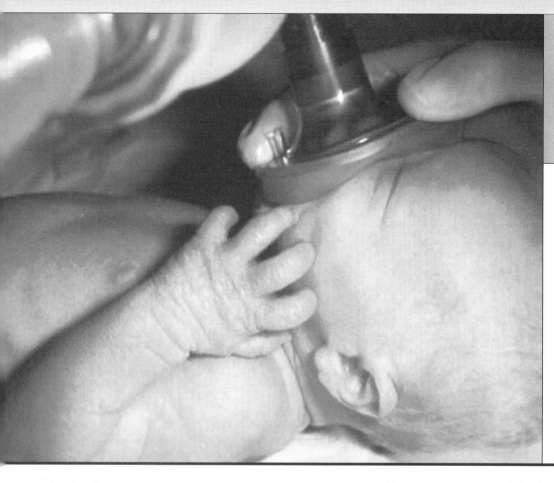

3

Premature Newborn with Cardio-pulmonary Depression

You arrive at a residence at 112 East Schweppe Street, where a father has just delivered his 34-week gestation daughter. The umbilical cord is still intact and the newborn, who has a weak cry, has cyanosis to the face, neck, and trunk. After quickly evaluating the newborn for signs of meconium, you perform the initial steps of resuscitation.

1. What are the initial steps of newborn resuscitation?

After completing your initial interventions, you perform a quick assessment of the newborn's cardiopulmonary status (**Table 3-1**). The mother, who is being comforted by her husband, tells you that this is her first baby.

Table 3-1 Rapid Cardiopulmonary Assessment

Airway and Breathing	Airway is patent (after suctioning); respirations, normal rate but irregular; adequate tidal volume
Heart Rate	90 beats/min and regular
Color	Peripheral and central cyanosis

2. When is management indicated for this newborn?

_____

_____

_____

_____

Following 30 seconds of treatment, you reassess the newborn and note that respirations have become shallow. Additionally, the newborn's heart rate is 50 beats/min and its trunk is becoming increasingly cyanotic. Your partner prepares for additional treatment.

3. How will you manage this newborn now?

_____

_____

_____

_____

The appropriate management is continued for the newborn. In addition, steps are taken to preserve the newborn's body heat. After 30 seconds of additional treatment, you reassess the newborn (**Table 3-2**). The mother, who remains conscious and alert, has been placed on 100% oxygen via nonrebreathing mask.

Table 3-2 Newborn Reassessment

Airway and Breathing	Intubated; ventilated at a rate of 40-60 breaths/min
Heart Rate	60 beats/min, weak and regular
Color	Peripheral and central cyanosis

A back-up crew of two paramedics arrives to provide assistance. Despite effective resuscitative efforts, the infant remains bradycardic and hypoxic. You and your partner agree that epinephrine is indicated. With difficulty, one of the assisting paramedics establishes a 26-gauge IV in the infant's antecubital vein. Blood is also obtained for a blood glucose reading

4. What is the appropriate dose and route for epinephrine in this newborn?

Following the administration of epinephrine, you reassess the newborn and find that her heart rate has increased to 90 beats/min. Chest compressions are therefore discontinued; however, positive-pressure ventilations are continued. An assisting paramedic advises you that the newborn's blood glucose reading is 40 mg/dL.

5. What additional treatment is indicated for this newborn?

Following additional treatment, the newborn's condition improves significantly. You reassess her heart rate and note that it is 120 beats/min. Your partner is continuing assisted ventilations; however, the infant is not resisting the ET tube. After clamping and cutting the umbilical cord, you quickly load mother and baby into the ambulance and proceed to a children's hospital located 10 miles away.

6. Why are premature newborns at higher risk for complications?

_____

_____

_____

_____

The newborn's condition continues to improve en route to the hospital. You continue thermal management, perform an ongoing assessment (**Table 3-3**), and call your radio report in to the receiving facility. En route, the placenta delivers and is appropriately cared for.

Table 3-3 Ongoing Assessment

Level of Activity	Conscious, good muscle tone
Airway and Breathing	Intubated (confirmed with capnometry); breath sounds, clear and equal bilaterally; ventilations provided as needed to maintain a heart rate of greater than 100 beats/min
Heart Rate	130 beats/min, strong and regular
Color	Peripheral cyanosis, centrally pink
Blood Glucose	90 mg/dL

You deliver the mother and baby to the hospital in stable condition. After additional assessment and treatment in the emergency department, the mother is admitted to the postpartum unit and the newborn is admitted to the neonatal ICU for additional evaluation and monitoring.

1. What are the initial steps of newborn resuscitation?

Following delivery of a newborn, a series of initial resuscitative steps are provided in order to facilitate the transition to extrauterine life. The extent of these initial steps depends on the findings of the postpartum evaluation (**Table 3-4**), which is rapidly performed immediately following birth.

Table 3-4 Postpartum Evaluation of the Newborn

Is the amniotic fluid clear of meconium?[1]

Is the newborn breathing or crying?

Does the newborn have good muscle tone?

Is the infant's color pink?[2]

Is this a term gestation?[3]

[1] Meconium, which has the consistency of tar, is the baby's first bowel movement, and should occur within the first 24 hours following birth. If meconium is present in the amniotic fluid, there is a chance that the newborn could have aspirated it. Treatment for meconium depends on the newborn's clinical presentation.

[2] Peripheral cyanosis (acrocyanosis) is a normal finding and may be present for several hours to a few days following birth. Central cyanosis (cyanotic face, neck, or trunk), however, is **not** normal and indicates the need for supplemental oxygen.

[3] Term gestation is considered to be from 37-42 weeks.

If the answer to **any** of the questions in **Table 3-4** is "no," then the newborn should be assumed to have respiratory depression, cardiovascular depression, or both, and in need of aggressive initial resuscitative steps (**Table 3-5**). Otherwise, the initial steps are mainly supportive and focus on providing warmth, maintaining a clear airway, and drying the newborn.

Table 3-5 Initial Steps of Newborn Resuscitation

Dry
- Vigorously dry the infant, paying particular attention to the head since it is proportionately large and emits a significant amount of heat.
  - If possible, cover the newborn's head with a towel or newborn hat.
- Vigorous drying of the newborn will often stimulate effective respirations.

Warm
- Ensure a warm resuscitation environment.
  - If in the ambulance, ensure that the heater is turned on.
  - If in a residence, turn on the central heat or provide some other source of adequate heat.
- Drying and warming should be performed simultaneously.

Position the newborn
- Place the newborn in a supine position with *slight* extension of the head or on its side to facilitate drainage of secretions (fetal lung fluid).
  - If the umbilical cord has not been clamped and cut, position the infant below the level of the perineum; this will prevent blood from draining back into the placenta from the infant.

Suction
- Suction the mouth first, then the nose.

Stimulation (Tactile)
- Flick the soles of the feet or briskly rub the lateral chest or back to stimulate effective breathing.

A useful mnemonic to assist you in remembering the initial steps of newborn resuscitation is to "**D**o **W**hat **P**robably **S**eems **S**imple" (**D**ry, **W**arm, **P**osition, **S**uction, **S**timulate). Following the initial steps of newborn resuscitation, a cardiopulmonary assessment is performed to determine the need for and extent of further resuscitation.

According to the American Academy of Pediatrics, nearly 90% of newborns are vigorous term babies that have clear amniotic fluid and effective breathing immediately following birth. Following clamping and cutting of the umbilical cord, they usually do not need to be separated from their mothers to provide further care.

2. When is management indicated for this newborn?

Following the initial steps of newborn resuscitation, a rapid cardiopulmonary assessment is performed, which focuses on three parameters: respiratory effort, heart rate, and color.

This infant is in need of *positive-pressure ventilations (PPV)*, as evidenced by the following clinical findings:

- **Heart rate of 90 beats/min**
  - Newborn bradycardia exists when the heart rate is less than 100 beats/min and is treated with PPV.
  - Provide PPV at a rate of 40 to 60 breaths/min for 30 seconds and then reassess the newborn's heart rate.

Other indications for PPV in the newborn include gasping respirations or apnea, cardiopulmonary arrest, and persistent central cyanosis despite the administration of blow-by oxygen.

Bradycardia in infants and children (including newborns) is almost always the result of hypoxia, not a cardiac event. Because they are very sensitive to oxygen, their heart rate usually responds quickly to PPV and 100% supplemental oxygen. To assess the newborn's heart rate, auscultate the heartbeat with a stethoscope (apical pulse), palpate the brachial pulse, or palpate the pulse at the base of the umbilical cord (**Figure 3-1**).

A useful method for calculating the newborn's heart rate is to count the number of pulsations in a 6-second time frame and multiply that number by 10. For example:

11 pulsations in 6 seconds × 10 = 110 beats/min

Irregular respirations are a normal finding in the newborn and, unless associated with reduced tidal volume (shallow breathing), bradypnea, or gasping, are not treated with PPV.

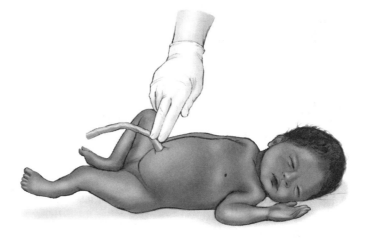

■ **Figure 3-1** Palpate for a pulse at the base of the umbilical cord.

The presence of central cyanosis alone (eg, normal heart rate and respirations) is treated initially with supplemental (blow-by) oxygen at 5 L/min via oxygen tubing or facemask. However, in the presence of bradycardia, central cyanosis is likely the result of significant hypoxemia and reinforces the need for PPV.

3. How will you manage this newborn now?

This newborn's condition is clearly deteriorating despite PPV with 100% oxygen. At this point, after ensuring effective bag-valve-mask ventilations (eg, adequate mask-to-face seal, good chest rise), the delivery of 100% oxygen, and a clear airway, you must now perform the following treatment interventions:

- **Chest compressions**
  - Chest compressions are indicated if the newborn's heart rate falls below 60 beats/min despite 30 seconds of effective PPV with 100% oxygen.
    - Perform chest compressions at a rate of 120 compressions/min at a depth that is approximately one-third of the anterior-posterior diameter of the newborn's chest.

You must avoid giving a compression and a ventilation simultaneously, as one will decrease the effectiveness of the other. Ventilations and compressions are therefore performed synchronously, with one ventilation given after every third compression. At this rate, a total of 30 breaths and 90 compressions will be performed each minute.

Profound newborn bradycardia (heart rate < 60 beats/min) indicates severely low blood-oxygen levels. This results in decreased myocardial contractility and a decreased amount of blood pumped to the lungs to pick up oxygen.

Chest compressions in the newborn are usually required only for a short period of time (30 to 60 seconds), until the myocardium recovers and resumes its ability to function adequately.

- **Endotracheal intubation**
  - During prolonged PPV with a bag-valve-mask device, the risk of gastric distention is very high; therefore, you should consider intubating the newborn. Intubation will also increase the effectiveness of delivered ventilations.
    - If intubation is not possible, consider inserting an orogastric tube to decompress the stomach.

There are many benefits to endotracheal intubation. It allows for the instillation of 100% oxygen directly into the lungs; it provides a route for certain resuscitative medications; and it virtually eliminates the risk of gastric distention.

During the course of a newborn resuscitation, endotracheal intubation can be considered at any point—especially if prolonged PPV is anticipated, chest compressions are being performed, or if certain medications need to be administered.

To avoid exacerbating newborn bradycardia and hypoxia, you must limit your intubation attempts to 20 seconds. Once you obtain a laryngoscopic view of the glottis, determine if the vocal cords are open or closed. If the cords are together (closed), do not touch them with the laryngoscope blade, as this may result in laryngospasm. If the cords do not open within 20 seconds, provide PPV for 30 to 60 seconds prior to reattempting intubation.

The appropriate-sized ET tube is determined by estimating the newborn's weight in grams (**Table 3-6**). However, you may also use the diameter of the newborn's little fingernail to estimate ET tube size. Only uncuffed ET tubes are used in newborns.

Table 3-6 ET Tube Size Based on the Newborn's Weight

Tube size	Weight	Gestational age
2.5 mm	< 1,000 g	< 28 weeks
3.0 mm	1,000-2,000 g	28-34 weeks
3.5 mm	2,000-3,000 g	34-38 weeks
3.5-4.0 mm	> 3,000 g	> 38 weeks

For premature newborns (less than 37 weeks or 5.5 lbs [2.5 kg]), use a size 0 blade; a size 1 blade should be used for term babies. Most clinicians advocate the use of a straight blade rather than a curved blade. Curved blades can be difficult to use in infants because their epiglottis is proportionately larger and much floppier. Additionally, curved blades are associated with a higher incidence of vagal-induced bradycardia.

4. What is the appropriate dose and route for epinephrine in this newborn?

IV administration of epinephrine is preferred over endotracheal administration. Since vascular access has been obtained, the following dose of epinephrine should be administered to the newborn:

- 0.01 to 0.03 mg/kg (0.1 to 0.3 mL/kg) of a 1:10,000 solution via rapid administration
  - Repeat this dose every 3 to 5 minutes as needed.

Epinephrine increases the rate (chronotropy) and force (inotropy) of cardiac contractions, as well as vasoconstriction, which will enhance cardiac and cerebral perfusion pressure.

Epinephrine is available in both 1:1,000 and 1:10,000 concentrations; however, only the 1:10,000 concentration should be used in newborns. Epinephrine 1:1,000 is too concentrated and thus too strong for use in newborns. Because newborns have a relatively fragile network of cerebral vasculature, strong doses of epinephrine may cause excessive vasoconstriction, resulting in a spontaneous intracranial hemorrhage. Additionally, using the 1:10,000 concentration will avoid the need to dilute the 1:1,000 concentration.

Atropine sulfate is rarely indicated in the newborn. Newborn bradycardia is most often the result of hypoxia, not parasympathetic nervous system stimulation. Therefore, atropine would be of no benefit. Additionally, if atropine is given in a dose of less than 0.1 mg, or if it is given too slowly, a paradoxical (reflex) bradycardia may occur.

Epinephrine is the preferred drug to treat severe newborn bradycardia because of its direct effect on the myocardium, which may need an adrenergic "boost" to help overcome the decreased contractility caused by hypoxia.

5. What additional treatment is indicated for this newborn?

This newborn's hypoglycemia has most likely contributed to her poor response to your resuscitation efforts. You must administer 10% dextrose (D_{10}) in the following dose:

- 2 mL/kg (0.1 g/mL concentration) via IV administration
  - Reassess blood glucose following administration and repeat the D_{10} (same dose) as needed.

Most ambulances do not carry D_{10}; therefore, you will have to dilute 50% dextrose (D_{50}) or 25% dextrose (D_{25}) to achieve the appropriate concentration. To convert D_{50} to D_{10}, simply dilute 10 mL of D_{50} (5 g) in 40 mL of normal saline. D_{25} and D_{50} are too concentrated for use in newborns and may result in hyperglycemia.

Newborns, especially when premature, have very limited glycogen stores. These limited glycogen stores are often rapidly depleted by not only the delivery process itself, but by the resuscitation that is sometimes needed. Additionally, the conversion of glycogen to glucose (glycogenolysis) is less efficient in premature newborns.

Newborn hypoglycemia may be difficult to recognize because the clinical signs are often subtle or nonspecific. The only presenting sign may be a poor response to resuscitation.

Prolonged hypoglycemia may cause permanent brain damage or even death; therefore, if a serum glucose reading of 40 mg/dL or less is documented in a depressed newborn, administer D_{10} without delay.

6. Why are premature newborns at higher risk for complications?

A premature newborn is one who is less than 37 weeks' gestation or who weighs less than 5.5 lbs (2.5 kg). Premature babies have anatomic and physiologic characteristics that are significantly different from term babies. Because of these differences, the premature newborn is at higher risk for the following complications following delivery:

- **Increased heat loss**
  - This is due to the premature newborn's thin, permeable skin and their large surface-area-to-body-mass ratio.
- **Difficult to ventilate**
  - The premature newborn's lungs may be deficient in pulmonary surfactant, resulting in increased alveolar surface tension.
- **Infection (sepsis)**
  - Compared to term babies, premature babies have even more underdeveloped immune systems.
- **Intracranial hemorrhage**
  - The premature newborn's cerebral capillaries are very fragile and may bleed during periods of stress (eg, resuscitation, hypoglycemia, hypoxia).
- **Hypovolemic shock**
  - Premature newborns have even less blood volume than term babies; therefore, even a minute amount of blood loss (eg, umbilical cord blood) may result in hypovolemic shock.
- **Hypoglycemia**
  - Due to limited glycogen stores and decreased glycogenolysis

During your assessment of a mother in labor, it is important to determine how far along she is in her pregnancy. If she is less than 37 weeks' gestation or ultrasound evaluation has estimated the fetal weight to be less than 5.5 lbs, you must be prepared to resuscitate the newborn following birth.

Summary

Most babies are born without complications, even in the prehospital setting. However, approximately 10% of newborns require resuscitation beyond the initial steps. The key to successful newborn resuscitation is anticipating the need for resuscitation and being prepared, both logistically and psychologically.

In addition to the initial steps of resuscitation, which are carried out on every newborn regardless of their appearance at birth, common interventions include oxygen administration and positive-pressure ventilations. Less common interventions include chest compressions, intubation, and medication administration. The "inverted pyramid" of newborn resuscitation (**Figure 3-2**) represents the most-to-least common interventions required in the resuscitation of the infant at birth.

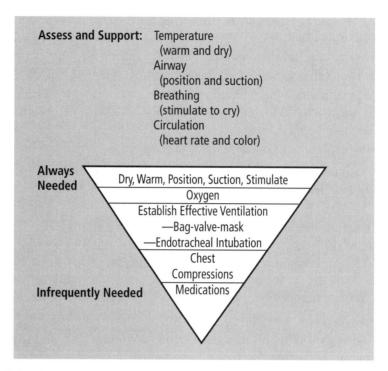

Assess and Support: Temperature
(warm and dry)
Airway
(position and suction)
Breathing
(stimulate to cry)
Circulation
(heart rate and color)

Always Needed

Dry, Warm, Position, Suction, Stimulate
Oxygen
Establish Effective Ventilation
—Bag-valve-mask
—Endotracheal Intubation
Chest
Compressions
Medications

Infrequently Needed

■ **Figure 3-2** The inverted pyramid of newborn resuscitation represents the frequency of interventions required during the resuscitation of an infant at birth. Source: American Heart Association.

The APGAR score is a measure of the effectiveness of interventions and should not be used to determine the need for and extent of resuscitation. Additionally, the first APGAR score is not evaluated until the newborn is 1 minute of age. Resuscitation, if needed, should commence within the first 30 seconds following birth. The need for resuscitation is therefore dependent on the infant's respiratory effort, heart rate, and color.

Following a successful newborn resuscitation, or if minimal resuscitation is needed, keep the newborn warm, maintain airway patency, clamp and cut the umbilical cord, and provide safe transport of the mother and baby to the hospital.

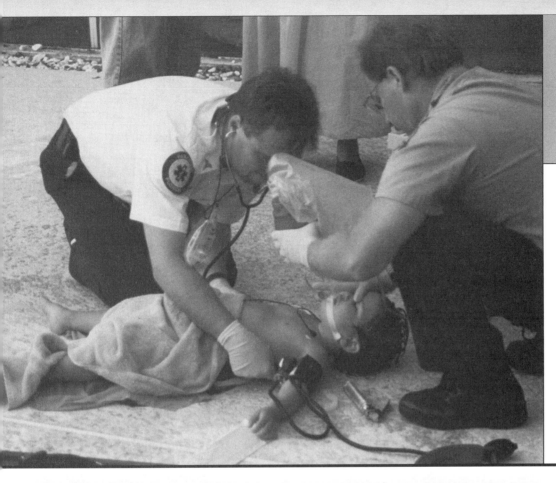

4-Year-Old Male Who Was Electrocuted

At 1:35 PM, a frantic mother calls 9-1-1, screaming that her 4-year-old son is "not breathing." The call is located at a residence at 556 West Kronkosky Street, which is approximately 5 miles from your station. An engine company and a paramedic supervisor are simultaneously dispatched to the scene.

Your unit and the engine company arrive at the scene simultaneously. You enter the residence and find the child lying supine and motionless on the living room floor. According to the mother, the child was electrocuted when he stuck a pin into an electrical outlet. The child is no longer in contact with the electrical socket; he is safe for you to touch. As your partner assumes manual in-line cervical spine stabilization, you perform an initial assessment (Table 4-1).

Table 4-1 Initial Assessment

Level of Consciousness	Unconscious and unresponsive
Mechanism of Injury	Electrocution
Airway and Breathing	Airway is patent, breathing is absent.
Circulation	No palpable carotid pulse, small arc-burn wound noted to left hand, no gross bleeding

1. What is your initial course of action?

_____

_____

_____

_____

After ensuring that nobody is touching the child, you assess his cardiac rhythm (**Figure 4-1**). The paramedic supervisor arrives to assist you with patient care.

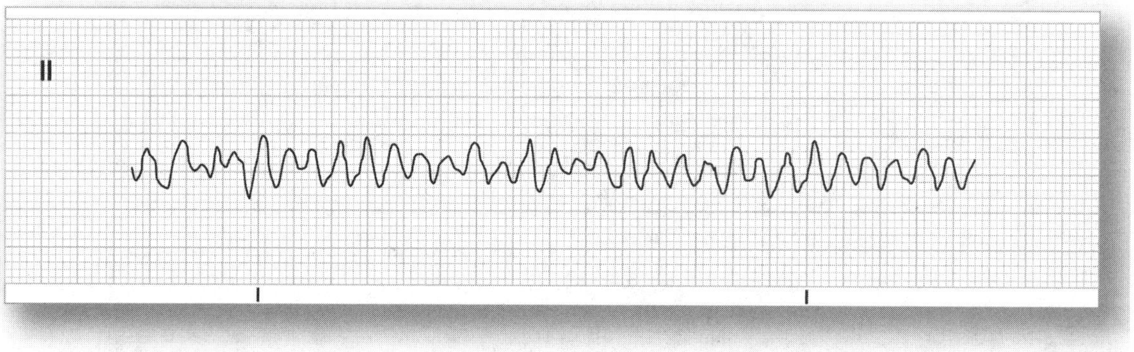

■ **Figure 4-1** The child's cardiac rhythm.

2. What is this child's cardiac rhythm? How will you treat it initially?

_____

_____

_____

Your initial interventions to treat the child's cardiac dysrhythmia are unsuccessful. After reconfirming pulselessness and apnea, you direct two fire fighters to initiate CPR and a third fire fighter to maintain cervical spine stabilization. Your partner prepares the intubation equipment as bag-valve-mask ventilations are continued. The paramedic supervisor establishes an IV line of normal saline in the child's antecubital fossa.

3. What is the first medication and dose that should be administered to this child?

_____

_____

_____

The appropriate initial medication has been administered to the child. After circulating the drug with CPR for 2 minutes, you reassess the child's cardiac rhythm. Noting that the cardiac rhythm is unchanged, you defibrillate the child at the appropriate energy setting. After preoxygenating the child, your partner proceeds with endotracheal intubation.

4. How does the child's airway anatomy affect endotracheal intubation?

_____

_____

_____

Your partner has placed the ET tube and has confirmed correct placement by auscultation of breath sounds and capnography. After securing the ET tube, ventilations are continued at the appropriate rate. Following your next defibrillation, which was unsuccessful, you consider antiarrhythmic therapy for this child.

5. What antiarrhythmic medications and doses are indicated for this child?

_____

_____

_____

After administering the appropriate antiarrhythmic, you circulate the drug with CPR for 2 minutes, and then reassess the cardiac rhythm. Following your next defibrillation, you observe a change in the child's cardiac rhythm (**Figure 4-2**).

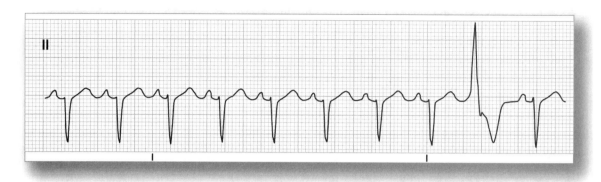

■ **Figure 4-2** The child's cardiac rhythm has changed.

Noting the change in the child's cardiac rhythm, you immediately reassess his condition (**Table 4-2**). Fire fighters have retrieved a cervical collar, head blocks, spine board, and the ambulance stretcher in preparation for transport to the hospital.

Table 4-2 Post-Resuscitation Reassessment

Level of Consciousness	Unconscious and unresponsive
Airway and Breathing	Intubated, ventilated at a rate of 20 breaths/min
Oxygen Saturation	95% (intubated and ventilated)
Circulation	Palpable femoral pulse at 100 beats/min; blood pressure, 70/40 mm Hg
ECG	Sinus rhythm with PVCs

Full spinal motion restriction precautions are taken and the child is quickly loaded into the ambulance. Rapid transport is begun to a hospital, which is located 15 miles away. En route, you perform additional interventions to further stabilize the child's condition.

6. What interventions should you perform while en route to the hospital?

The child's condition has improved following additional treatment. He has occasional respirations, is semiconscious, and his blood pressure has improved. After performing an ongoing assessment (**Table 4-3**), you call your radio report to the receiving facility with an estimated time of arrival of 5 minutes.

Table 4-3 Ongoing Assessment

Level of Consciousness	Semiconscious, beginning to resist the ET tube
Airway and Breathing	Intubated, occasional respirations (assisted)
Oxygen Saturation	97% (intubated and ventilated)
Circulation	Radial pulse, 120 beats/min and regular; blood pressure, 90/60 mm Hg
ECG	Normal sinus rhythm

After administering midazolam (Versed) (0.05–0.2 mg/kg) to the child for sedation, he becomes more compliant with the ET tube. You deliver the child to the emergency department, where the attending physician immediately greets you. Following additional assessment and treatment in the emergency department, the child is admitted to the pediatric ICU. He later recovers and is discharged home.

CASE STUDY ANSWERS AND SUMMARY

1. What is your initial course of action?

Once cardiac arrest is confirmed by determining pulselessness and apnea, your priority is to *assess the need for defibrillation*. Rapid cardiac rhythm analysis is performed by placing the appropriate-sized defibrillation pads (also called "multi-pads") on the child's chest, or by using the defibrillator paddles. Determining the correct paddle size is based on the child's age and weight (**Table 4-4**).

Table 4-4 Determining the Correct Defibrillation Paddle Size

Paddle size	Age	Weight[1]
4.5 cm (pediatric)	< 12 months	< 10 kg (< 22 lbs)
8.0–10 cm (adult)	> 12 months	> 10 kg (> 22 lbs)

[1] If an infant weighs more than 10 kg, even if he or she is under 12 months of age, use the 8.0–10 cm paddles. Conversely, if a child weighs less than 10 kg, even if he or she is older than 12 months of age, use the 4.5 cm paddles.

In infants up to 12 months of age *or* who weigh less than 10 kg (22 lbs), anterior paddle placement is recommended (**Figure 4-3**). In children over 12 months of age *or* who weigh more than 10 kg, use either anterior paddle placement or place the child on his/her side and use the anterior-posterior placement method (**Figure 4-4**). If spinal motion restriction is indicated, anterior paddle placement should be used .

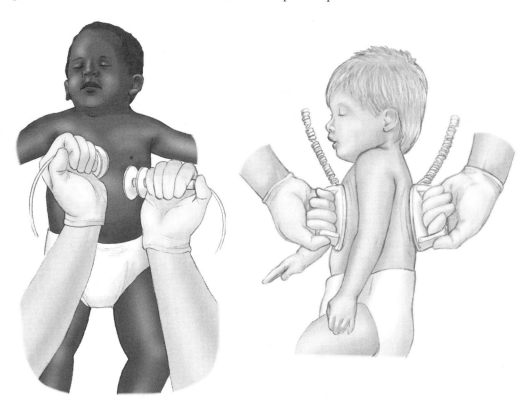

■ **Figure 4-3** Site for paddles on the anterior chest wall.

■ **Figure 4-4** Site for paddles with child on side and paddles placed in the anterior-posterior position.

If you are using pediatric defibrillation pads, apply the pads directly to the skin and ensure that no air pockets exist between the pads and the chest wall. Place the sternum pad on the anterior chest wall to the right of the upper sternum, inferior to the clavicle; place the apex pad on the midclavicular line at the level of the xiphoid process (**Figure 4-5**).

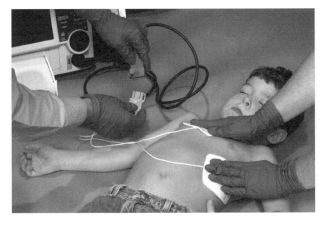

Figure 4-5 Appropriate placement for pediatric defibrillation pads.

According to the 2005 Emergency Cardiac Care (ECC) guidelines, data has shown that AEDs can safely and effectively be used in children 1 to 8 years of age. It is recommended that the AED have both a high specificity in recognizing pediatric shockable rhythms (ie, V-fib, pulseless V-tach) and a pediatric dose-attenuating system to reduce the amount of energy delivered by the AED. If, however, an AED with a pediatric dose-attenuating system is not available, a standard AED should be used. Currently, there is insufficient data to support the use of AEDs in infants (< 1 year of age).

2. What is the child's cardiac rhythm? How will you treat it initially?

This child is in *ventricular fibrillation* (**Figure 4-6**). The rhythm is characterized by a chaotic baseline, with no discernable waves or intervals. Ventricular fibrillation (V-fib) is caused by multiple ectopic ventricular foci, which cause the heart to "quiver." There is no pulse or cardiac output associated with V-fib.

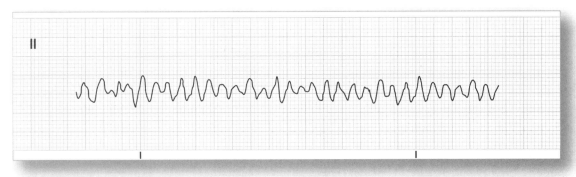

Figure 4-6 Ventricular fibrillation.

Cardiac arrest in infants and children is typically the result of respiratory failure and often presents with a bradydysrhythmia or asystole. However, ventricular arrhythmias, such as V-fib and pulseless V-tach can occur, and are usually the result of non-respiratory factors, such as electrocution, myocarditis, and congenital heart defects.

Regardless of the cause of the ventricular arrhythmia, the initial treatment is the same as that for an adult and just as critical—early defibrillation!

Defibrillate the pediatric patient in V-fib one time at 2 joules/kg, followed immediately by CPR. After 2 minutes of CPR, reassess the cardiac rhythm. If V-fib persists, defibrillate again with 4 joules/kg, followed immediately by CPR. It is important to minimize any delays or interruptions in CPR; as soon as the child has been defibrillated, immediately resume CPR.

Do not delay defibrillation in the child to obtain venous access or to place an endotracheal tube. According to the American Heart Association, the chance of survival decreases by approximately 7% to 10% for each minute that V-fib persists. **Table 4-5** lists the steps to take in order to maximize defibrillation success.

Table 4-5 Maximizing Successful Defibrillation

Use the appropriate paddle size.   • Based on age and weight
Ensure full contact with the skin.   • Partial contact will cause skin burns and reduce the effectiveness of the defibrillation.
Use a conductive medium.   • Pregelled pediatric pads or conductive paste/gel   • Apply conductive gel to the defibrillation paddles, if used.

3. What is the first medication and dose that should be administered to this child?

The first medication that should be administered to this child is *epinephrine*. The dose, however, depends upon the route by which the drug will be administered:

- **Intravenous or intraosseous**
  - 0.01 mg/kg (0.1 mL/kg) of a 1:10,000 solution

- **Endotracheal administration**
  - 0.1 mg/kg (0.1 mL/kg) of a 1:1,000 solution
    - Flush with 5 mL of normal saline

Epinephrine should be repeated every 3 to 5 minutes in the doses stated above. The maximum dose of epinephrine given via the IV/IO route is 1 mg; 10 mg if given via the ET tube. Circulate the drug with CPR for 2 minutes and then reassess the cardiac rhythm. Defibrillate at 4 joules/kg if V-fib persists, followed by immediate resumption of CPR.

Higher subsequent doses of epinephrine may be required for special resuscitation situations, in which greater adrenergic stimulation is needed. These situations include, among others, beta-blocker overdose (eg, Lopressor, Inderal) and status asthmaticus. Contact medical control as needed regarding higher epinephrine dosing.

Epinephrine stimulates both alpha and beta adrenergic receptors. However, during cardiac arrest, the main benefit of epinephrine comes from its alpha-induced vasoconstrictive effects, which enhance cerebral and coronary perfusion. Epinephrine is therefore a pharmacological adjunct to CPR.

4. How does the child's airway anatomy affect endotracheal intubation?

Although the airway maneuvers and indications for employing those maneuvers in infants and children are no different than in adults, there are several anatomical differences in children that are important to consider, especially when performing endotracheal intubation.

When placing the laryngoscope in the child's mouth, the first thing you are likely to notice is the size of his or her tongue, which is proportionately larger than the adult's (**Figure 4-7**). This, in combination with a smaller mandible, increases the incidence of positional airway obstruction. Therefore, in between intubation attempts, when ventilating with a bag-valve-mask device, it is critical to correctly position the child's head. Padding underneath the child's head is often necessary in order to maintain the head in a neutral position.

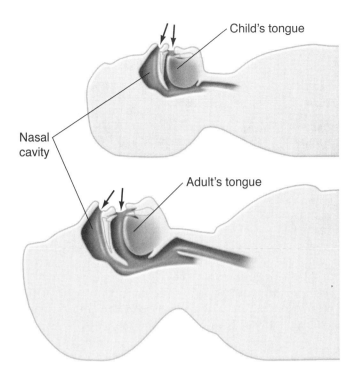

Child's tongue

Nasal cavity

Adult's tongue

■ **Figure 4-7** In children, the tongue is proportionately larger than it is in adults.

A child's epiglottis is floppier, longer, and more U-shaped than an adult's; therefore, it must be lifted or positioned out of the way in order to obtain a laryngoscopic view of the vocal cords (**Figure 4-8**). A straight blade is generally preferred when intubating children because of the ease with which it lifts the epiglottis and exposes the vocal cords.

The trachea in a child is shorter, smaller, and narrower than in an adult, and it is positioned more anteriorly and superiorly. Because of the small diameter of the child's trachea, an uncuffed ET tube should be used in children younger than 10 years of age.

The cricoid ring, located in the subglottic region (below the vocal cords), is the narrowest portion of the child's airway (**Figure 4-9**). In general, the subglottic airway in a child is more funnel-shaped as opposed to the straight tube in an adult, thus making a cuffed ET tube less necessary for occluding the trachea and allowing adequate positive-pressure ventilations to occur. Additionally, the developing cartilage of the cricoid ring could potentially be injured by inflation of a cuffed ET tube.

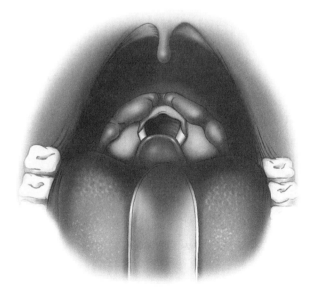

■ **Figure 4-8** A child's epiglottis is floppier, longer, and more U-shaped than an adult's.

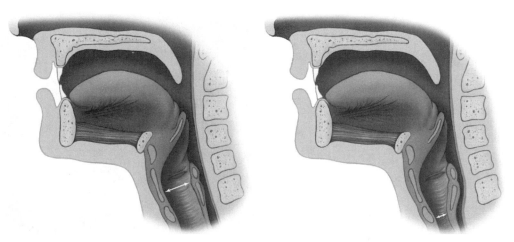

■ **Figure 4-9** The narrowest portion of the pediatric airway is at the cricoid ring.

Selecting the appropriate-sized ET tube and inserting the tube to the appropriate depth are critical aspects of pediatric endotracheal intubation (**Table 4-6**).

Table 4-6 Pediatric ET Tube Sizes and Depths of Insertion

Age	ET Tube Size (mm)	Insertion Depth (cm)
Premature infant	2.0-2.5 uncuffed	6.0-8.0
Term newborn	3.0-3.5 uncuffed	8.0-9.0
Infant to 1 year	3.5-4.0 uncuffed	9.5-2.0
Toddler (2-4 years)	4.5-5.0 uncuffed	12.0-15.0
Preschool (5-6 years)	5.0-5.5 uncuffed	15.0-16.5
School age (6-10 years)	5.5-6.5 uncuffed	16.5-19.5
School age (10-12 years)	6.5 cuffed	19.5
Adolescent	7.0-8.0 cuffed	20.0-23.0

Other methods to use when selecting the appropriately sized ET tube for the pediatric patient include the length-based resuscitation tape or anatomic clues, such as the diameter of the child's little fingernail or external nares. For children over 1 year of age, either of the following formulae can be used to determine the correct-sized ET tube:

■ **Formula 1: Age (in years) ÷ 4 + 4**
  • *4 (age in years) ÷ 4 + 4 = 5.0-mm ET tube*
■ **Formula 2: Age (in years) + 16 ÷ 4**
  • *4 (age in years) + 16 ÷ 4 = 5.0-mm ET tube*

To determine the appropriate depth of insertion (cm) of the ET tube, use one of the following formulae, based on the child's age:

■ **Depth of insertion (cm) = age (in years) ÷ 2 + 12**
  • For children older than 2 years of age
■ **Depth of insertion (cm) = ET tube internal diameter (mm) × 3**
  • For children of any age

5. What antiarrhythmic medications and doses are indicated for this child?

According to the American Academy of Pediatrics, you should administer **one** of the following antiarrhythmic medications to treat a child with shock-refractory V-fib or pulseless V-tach:

- Amiodarone (Cordarone) 5 mg/kg via IV or IO administration
  - Repeat up to 15 mg/kg
  - Maximum total dose is 300 mg
- Lidocaine (Xylocaine) 1 mg/kg[1] via IV or IO administration
  - Repeat dose at 0.5 to 1 mg/kg
  - Maximum total dose is 100 mg

[1]Administer 2 to 3 mg/kg via the ET tube, followed by a 5 mL flush of normal saline.

Amiodarone and lidocaine are both associated with prolongation of the QT interval; therefore, concurrent use of these medications is not recommended by the American Academy of Pediatrics.

6. What interventions should you perform while en route to the hospital?

Post-resuscitation management is a critical aspect in the care of any patient who has been resuscitated from cardiac arrest. Certain interventions must be performed in order to stabilize the patient and prevent the recurrence of cardiac arrest. En route to the hospital, the following interventions should be performed:

- **Reassess ET tube placement.**
  - Reauscultate breath sounds bilaterally and over the epigastrium.
  - Reassess the end-tidal CO_2 detector or attach a digital capnometer.

A critical intervention in the intubated patient is to *frequently* reassess placement of the ET tube. This is especially true after any major patient move, such as when the patient is moved from the ground to the stretcher or after the patient is loaded into the ambulance. A dislodged ET tube is not always so easily replaced. ET tube placement should be confirmed by *at least* two methods.

First, you should reauscultate breath sounds bilaterally and reauscultate over the epigastrium. Additionally, you should reassess the end-tidal CO_2 (ETCO$_2$) detector for the appropriate color change. Note, however, that the ETCO$_2$ detector may not be reliable in patients who are severely hypoxic and acidotic. Pediatric ETCO$_2$ detectors should be used in children who weigh 15 kg or less.

The esophageal detector device (EDD) should only be used in children with a perfusing rhythm (eg, non-cardiac arrest) who weigh more than 20 kg. Because the tracheal walls in children collapse more easily and there is a reduced volume of exhaled air, the bulb or syringe may not fill quickly, producing a false indication that the ET tube is in the esophagus when it is actually in the trachea.

Electronic waveform capnometry is an excellent way of confirming correct ET tube placement because it quantifies exhaled CO_2 with instantaneous, accurate data. This is especially useful in the back of a moving ambulance, where breath sounds are often difficult, if not impossible, to auscultate. The capnometer uses a connector (T-piece) that is placed in-line between the capnometer and ET tube. Along with your clinical assessment, the capnometer will not only assist you in determining correct ET tube placement, but it can also help determine whether the patient's condition is improving or deteriorating over time.

Like the ETCO$_2$ detector, electronic waveform capnometry is a less specific indicator of ET tube placement in patients with severe hypoxia and acidosis.

- **Blood pressure support**

Hypotension is commonly observed following resuscitation as the myocardium attempts to recover from cardiac arrest. Untreated hypotension can result in renal failure, brain damage, and other negative effects. Initial treatment for post-resuscitation hypotension should include a 20-mL/kg bolus of normal saline or lactated Ringer's solution. If hypotension persists, consider administering one of the following medications:

- Epinephrine (Adrenalin) 0.1–1 µg/kg/min

Epinephrine, an endogenous (naturally-occurring) catecholamine, is a potent inotrope that is typically infused at a rate sufficient to increase systemic vascular resistance and therefore blood pressure.

- Dopamine (Intropin) 2–20 µg/kg/min

Dopamine is also an endogenous catecholamine used to treat, among other conditions, fluid-refractory hypotension following resuscitation. To increase blood pressure and improve perfusion, start the infusion at 5 µg/kg/min and increase it as needed up to 20 µg/kg/min.

- Dobutamine (Dobutrex) 2–20 µg/kg/min

Dobutamine is a synthetic catecholamine that primarily affects beta$_1$ adrenergic receptors, resulting in increased contractility (inotropy). Additionally, dobutamine reduces systemic vascular resistance (afterload), thus decreasing left ventricular workload. Dobutamine may be particularly useful in treating hypotension and decreased cardiac output secondary to poor myocardial function (eg, after cardiac arrest).

Sympathomimetic drugs (eg, epinephrine, dopamine, dobutamine) can cause an increase in myocardial oxygen demand and consumption. It is therefore critical to perform frequent cardiopulmonary assessments in the child if these medications are used in the management of post-resuscitation hypotension.

- ■ Antiarrhythmic infusion

After ensuring continued airway patency and stabilizing the child's blood pressure, you must turn your attention to preventing the recurrence of cardiac arrest. Administer a maintenance infusion of the antiarrhythmic drug that aided in the resuscitation.

The maintenance infusion dose of lidocaine for children is 20–50 µg/kg/min. If it has been greater than 15 minutes since the last bolus dose of lidocaine, administer another bolus of 1 mg/kg prior to initiating the maintenance infusion. This will maintain a therapeutic blood level of the drug.

Amiodarone maintenance infusions are not recommended by the American Academy of Pediatrics for use in children. If the V-fib recurs in the child, immediately defibrillate with the previously successful energy setting and then administer another amiodarone bolus of 5 mg/kg.

Summary

Cardiac arrest in children typically presents with a bradydysrhythmia or asystole and is most often the result of respiratory failure. However, in the child with an otherwise healthy heart, V-fib or pulseless V-tach can occur, and is typically the result of factors such as electrocution, myocarditis, or a congenital heart defect.

The treatment algorithm for pediatric V-fib and pulseless V-tach is essentially the same as it is for the adult, with the exception of the obviously smaller drug doses. Early defibrillation, as with the adult patient, is just as critical in children with V-fib or pulseless V-tach. Defibrillation must not be delayed by interventions such as IV therapy or endotracheal intubation. Survival rates decrease by approximately 7% to 10% for each minute that these lethal ventricular arrhythmias persist.

Following successful resuscitation, frequent cardiopulmonary assessments should be performed, and hemodynamic stability achieved as soon as possible. This includes IV crystalloid boluses and inotropic agents for hypotension, and an antiarrhythmic infusion to prevent recurrent cardiac arrest. If V-fib recurs, immediately defibrillate the child with the previously successful energy setting.

If the cardiac arrest is associated with a traumatic event, full spinal motion restriction precautions (eg, spinal immobilization) should be taken.

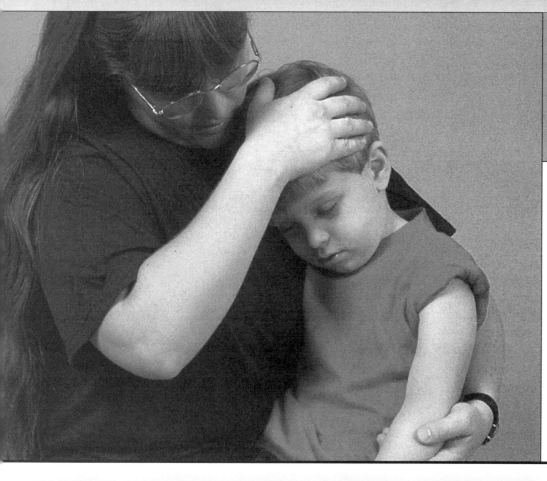

3-Year-Old Male with a Seizure

At 8:50 PM, you are dispatched to a residence at 435 Phil Wilson Street for a 3-year-old male who is having a seizure. Your response time to the scene is approximately 15 minutes, so you ask the dispatcher to send a first responder unit to the scene.

You enter the residence and find an ill-appearing child sitting on his mother's lap. He is conscious, crying, and clinging to his mother. As you perform an initial assessment (**Table 5-1**), the child's mother tells you that her son has been ill for the past 12 hours. Then he suddenly stopped responding to her and had a convulsion.

Table 5-1 Initial Assessment

Level of Consciousness	Conscious, crying, clinging to mom
Chief Complaint	Apparent seizure
Airway and Breathing	Airway is patent; respirations, increased and unlabored.
Circulation	Radial pulse, rapid and regular; skin, flushed and warm; capillary refill, 2 seconds

1. What are common causes of fever in children?

_____

_____

_____

_____

Your partner hands the mother an oxygen mask to hold near the child's face. The mother tells you that she gave her son acetaminophen about 45 minutes ago, shortly before the convulsion. You perform a focused history and physical examination (**Table 5-2**) with information gathered from the mother.

Table 5-2 Focused History and Physical Examination	
Description of the Episode	"He was crying, and then he suddenly stopped. His eyes rolled back and his whole body began to shake."
Duration	"He was shaking for about 2 minutes."
Associated Symptoms	"He has been running a fever for the past 12 hours."
Evidence of Trauma	None
Blood Glucose	102 mg/dL
Fever	101.5°F (axillary)
Interventions Prior to EMS Arrival	"I gave him some acetaminophen about 45 minutes ago."

2. What is the pathophysiology of a febrile seizure?

_____

_____

_____

_____

You obtain baseline vital signs and a SAMPLE history (**Table 5-3**). The child, who is still sitting on his mother's lap, is relatively cooperative. Your partner explains the need for transport to the hospital. The mother agrees, and asks that you transport her son to the hospital where his pediatrician practices, which is located 10 miles away.

Table 5-3 Baseline Vital Signs and SAMPLE History

Blood Pressure	80/50 mm Hg
Pulse	140 beats/min, strong and regular
Capillary Refill	2 seconds
Respirations	40 breaths/min; unlabored; adequate tidal volume
Oxygen Saturation	98% (on blow-by oxygen)
Signs and Symptoms	Fever, seizure, irritable
Allergies	None
Medications	None prescribed; one dose of acetaminophen given by mother
Pertinent Past History	None
Last Oral Intake	Lunch, approximately 8 hours ago
Events Leading to Present Illness	According to mother: "He had been running a fever, and then suddenly stopped responding to me and had a convulsion."

3. What additional treatment is indicated for this child?

After removing some of the child's clothing to keep him cool, the mother carries her son to the ambulance. You secure the child on the stretcher and begin transport. The mother is secured on the bench seat next to the stretcher. En route to the hospital, you perform an ongoing assessment (**Table 5-4**) while monitoring the child for further seizure activity.

Table 5-4 Ongoing Assessment

Level of Consciousness	Conscious, crying, clinging to mom
Airway and Breathing	Airway remains patent; respirations, 34 breaths/min and unlabored
Oxygen Saturation	98% (on blow-by oxygen)
Blood Pressure	Unable to obtain; the child will not cooperate.
Pulse	120 beats/min, strong and regular
Capillary Refill	1-2 seconds
Temperature	100.2°F (axillary)

4. What should you do if this child develops a prolonged seizure?

_____

_____

_____

_____

5. What is the appropriate care for the postictal child?

_____

_____

_____

You notice that the child is sweating—a sign that the fever is dissipating. The child is delivered to the emergency department and you give your verbal report to the charge nurse. Further assessment by the physician rules out serious causes of the seizure. The child is diagnosed with acute otitis media, is given ibuprofen and a prescribed antibiotic, and is discharged home with instructions to follow up with his pediatrician.

1. What are common causes of fever in children?

Fever occurs when the body's temperature increases above its normal baseline. Although the normal body temperature varies from person to person, it is usually around 98.6°F (37.0°C)

Fever is analogous to sinus tachycardia—it is a sign of an underlying problem, rather than a problem itself. Fever-causing agents, called pyrogens, are produced by the immune system in response to an invading or spreading organism. Fever, or pyrexia, is therefore a protective mechanism of the body to fight off infection. Once the underlying cause is treated (eg, infection), the number of circulating pyrogens decreases, and the fever dissipates.

Fever in children is most commonly the result of a viral or bacterial infection, usually of the respiratory tract or ears (**Table 5-5**). However, there are other causes of fever in children, some of which can be life-threatening. Therefore, the paramedic must carefully assess the febrile child and search for clues that suggest a serious underlying illness.

Table 5-5 Common Causes of Fever in Children

Upper or lower respiratory tract infections
- Croup
- Bronchiolitis
- Pneumonia
- Pharyngitis

Ear infections
- Otitis media (middle ear)
  - Most common
  - Usually associated with an upper respiratory tract infection
- Otitis externa (outer ear)

Central nervous system infections, such as meningitis and encephalitis, can cause fever in children as well. Meningitis is an infection and inflammation of the meninges surrounding the brain and spinal cord; encephalitis is an infection and inflammation of the brain. Meningitis and encephalitis are potentially life-threatening infections that can result in massive septic shock, seizures, brain damage, or even death.

Noninfectious causes of fever in children include salicylate overdose (aspirin), environmental hyperthermia (heatstroke), reactions to contaminated IV fluids or medications (pyrogenic reaction), and hypo- or hyperglycemia.

Fever is classified as being low-grade (100.0°F to 102.2°F) or high-grade (> 102.2°F) in children more than 3 months of age; however, unless associated with massive sepsis (eg, meningitis), or other life-threatening conditions, fever alone is usually not dangerous to the child.

2. What is the pathophysiology of a febrile seizure?

A febrile seizure occurs when fever suddenly develops, or when the already febrile child experiences a sudden fever spike. It is not necessarily how high the fever gets that causes the seizure, but rather how quickly it gets there.

Rapid elevations in body temperature interfere with normal hypothalamic function and normal impulse transmission in the brain, resulting in a massive and chaotic discharge of neurons. This massive neuronic discharge manifests as a seizure.

Most seizures in children are due to fever alone and are usually not associated with a serious underlying illness. However, because certain serious illnesses such as meningitis also present with fever and seizures, the diagnosis of a febrile seizure cannot be made in the prehospital setting. Therefore, a physician in the emergency department must evaluate any child with fever and seizures. *Fever with a seizure is clinically significant and is not the same as a febrile seizure.*

Most febrile seizures occur in children between 6 months and 5 years of age, with a history of fever. However, there is usually not a past history of seizure activity.

The seizure itself is usually a generalized seizure, characterized by tonic-clonic motor activity, in which the body alternates between muscular rigidity and flaccidity. Many febrile seizures are not followed by a postictal period. However, if a postictal period occurs, it is usually short-lived, with the child quickly regaining full neurological function.

Febrile seizures are categorized as being simple or complex (**Table 5-6**). Most febrile seizures are simple and occur in otherwise healthy children without a history of seizures.

Table 5-6 Simple and Complex Febrile Seizures

Simple febrile seizure
- Caused by a sudden onset of fever or a rapid increase in body temperature
- Tonic-clonic motor activity occurs, but is generally of a short duration.
- Absent or brief postictal period
- Child is otherwise healthy, without a history of nonfebrile seizures.
  - There may be a history of prior febrile seizures.

Complex febrile seizure
- Occurs as the result of persistent fever
- May present as a complex partial seizure:
  - Seizures to one part of the body, such as one arm or one leg
  - May be preceded by an aura (eg, strange taste or odor, strange feeling)
  - Complex partial seizures may progress to generalized seizures.
- Postictal period is usually prolonged.
- Seizure occurs more than once in a 24-hour period.
- A greater risk of developing status epilepticus

In the vast majority of cases, the child with a simple febrile seizure will have stopped seizing prior to EMS arrival at the scene. The child is usually conscious, crying, and febrile; however, they are usually hemodynamically stable.

3. What additional treatment is indicated for this child?

Since this child is hemodynamically stable, management should include supportive care and transport to the hospital, while monitoring for the development of another seizure. Continue to administer blow-by oxygen, unless the child becomes agitated and resistant to it. Also, in children older than 3 months of age with a fever greater than 101.2°F, simple cooling measures can be employed, such as removing clothing to allow for passive cooling.

Avoid cold water baths or fans to lower the child's body temperature (active cooling), as these measures may cause the child to shiver. Shivering is the body's way of producing heat, which in an already febrile child may precipitate another seizure.

The tachycardia and tachypnea that this child is experiencing is likely the result of the fever itself rather than hypovolemia. The presence of radial pulses and normal capillary refill time also rules out significant hypovolemia and shock. Therefore, IV therapy is not necessary at this point and will likely only agitate the child.

Febrile seizures are a terrifying event for the parent or caregiver to witness. Provide reassurance to the child's mother by explaining to her that transport to the hospital is necessary to rule out other causes of the seizure, and that the fever alone will not harm her child.

4. What should you do if this child develops a prolonged seizure?

Febrile seizures are rarely associated with status epilepticus. Status epilepticus occurs when the seizure is prolonged (> 20 minutes) or if two or more seizures occur in a row without an intervening period of alertness, muscle tone, or interactiveness. Permanent brain damage or death can occur as the result of status epilepticus, and is usually the result of prolonged hypoxia. Therefore, treatment is aimed at ensuring adequate oxygenation and ventilation, and terminating the seizure. Prehospital management for the actively seizing child includes the following:

- **Obtain and maintain a patent airway.**
  - As with the adult patient, do not attempt to pry the child's mouth open, as this may result in broken teeth, soft tissue trauma, and oropharyngeal bleeding.
  - Consider inserting a nasopharyngeal airway to assist in maintaining airway patency.
  - Suction oral secretions as necessary.
- Administer 100% supplemental oxygen (pediatric nonrebreathing mask).
  - Assist ventilations with a bag-valve-mask device if the child is breathing inadequately, is cyanotic, or has an oxygen saturation of less than 90% despite supplemental oxygen therapy.
- **Endotracheal intubation is generally contraindicated during a seizure and is almost always impossible to perform due to clenching of the teeth (trismus).**
- **Protect from further injury.**
  - Loosen restrictive clothing.
  - Do not physically restrain the child.
    - The tetanic muscle spasms that occur during a seizure can result in long bone fractures if the patient is physically restrained.
- **Anticonvulsant therapy**

Benzodiazepines are the first-line drugs used to terminate seizures in the prehospital setting. IV therapy is usually not necessary in the actively seizing child, because benzodiazepines can be given via the intramuscular (IM) or rectal route. Administer one of the following medications, according to locally established protocols or direct medical control:

- **Diazepam (Valium)**
  - Rectal: 0.5 mg/kg initially; repeat at 0.25 mg/kg every 10 to 15 minutes, up to three doses; maximum single dose is 10 mg.
  - IV or IO: 0.1 mg/kg; maximum dose is 4 mg.

Diazepam has a rapid onset of action; however, its anticonvulsant effects are relatively short. Therefore, additional dosing may be required within 10 to 20 minutes following the initial dose. Diazepam is not well-absorbed through muscle tissue and may cause muscle irritation; therefore, it should not be given via the IM route.

A major advantage of using diazepam is that it can be given via the rectal route. In infants and children, IV access can be difficult to obtain, and repeated attempts only delay pharmacological termination of the seizure. Diazepam is a lipid-soluble benzodiazepine that is rapidly absorbed across the rectal mucosa (**Figure 5-1**) and will terminate most seizures without the need for further treatment. The onset of action of rectally administered diazepam is approximately 2 to 5 minutes.

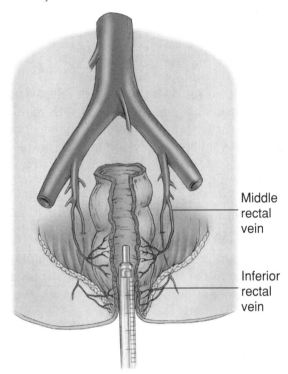

Middle rectal vein

Inferior rectal vein

■ **Figure 5-1** Diazepam is rapidly absorbed across the rectal mucosa and will terminate most seizures without the need for further treatment.

■ **Midazolam (Versed)**
  • 0.05 to 0.15 mg/kg via IV, IO, or IM injection

The onset of action of IM midazolam is approximately 15 minutes—only slightly shorter than if given via IV. Because IM midazolam usually lasts for up to 6 hours, repeat dosing in the prehospital setting is usually not necessary.

Lorazepam (Ativan) is also a commonly used benzodiazepine in the treatment of seizures. Lorazepam is similar to diazepam; however, its anticonvulsant effects last longer. Disadvantages of lorazepam are that it must be refrigerated and its shelf life is only about 90 days. The pediatric dose for lorazepam is 0.05 to 0.15 mg/kg via IV, IM, or IO administration.

Benzodiazepines, although to a lesser degree than more powerful CNS depressants (eg, opiates), can cause CNS depression, including hypoventilation, hypotension, and bradycardia. If this occurs, assisted ventilations will be necessary to restore adequate minute volume. If administering a benzodiazepine via the IV route, always give the medication slowly. Flumazenil (Romazicon), a benzodiazepine receptor antagonist, can be given to reverse the CNS depressant effects of benzodiazepines; however, it is not commonly carried in the prehospital setting. If your EMS system does carry flumazenil, follow local protocols or contact medical regarding the appropriate pediatric dose.

5. What is the appropriate care for the postictal child?

As previously discussed, the vast majority of febrile seizures will have stopped prior to EMS arrival at the scene. The postictal phase, which is more common with complex febrile seizures, is characterized by abnormal appearance, sleepiness, irritability, and decreased interactiveness, and may last only a few minutes or as long as a few hours.

During the postictal phase, provide supportive care, such as ensuring continued airway patency, oropharyngeal suctioning as needed, and administering supplemental oxygen.

If a benzodiazepine was administered to terminate the seizure, closely monitor the child for signs of CNS depression, and be prepared to support ventilations with a bag-valve-mask device.

Summary

Febrile seizures occur when the child suddenly develops a fever, or when an already febrile child experiences an abrupt fever spike. Febrile seizures are the most common type of seizure that you will encounter in the pediatric patient. Most febrile seizures occur in children between 6 months and 5 years of age, with a history of fever. Viral or bacterial infections are common underlying causes of fever in children, with middle ear infections (otitis media) being the most common.

For obvious reasons, the parent or caregiver becomes frightened and calls 9-1-1 for assistance. In the vast majority of cases, the seizure will have stopped prior to EMS arrival at the scene.

Because seizures and fever can occur with life-threatening conditions (eg, meningitis), the diagnosis of a febrile seizure requires physician evaluation in the emergency department. In the field, the paramedic must perform a careful assessment in order to identify signs and symptoms of a more severe underlying problem.

Prehospital management for the child post-seizure is mainly supportive, to include the administration of blow-by oxygen and removal of clothing to allow for passive cooling. Submersing the child in water or taking other measures to actively lower body temperature are not advisable, as these actions may cause shivering, which could cause an abrupt rise in body temperature and precipitate another seizure.

If the child is actively seizing, immediately ensure a patent airway and administer supplemental oxygen. Ventilatory support will be necessary if the child is breathing inadequately or is experiencing other signs of respiratory failure (eg, cyanosis, SaO_2 less than 90%). The seizure must then be terminated pharmacologically, using a benzodiazepine drug such as diazepam, midazolam, or lorazepam.

Care for the postictal child involves supportive care, such as continuing oxygen therapy and close monitoring for the development of another seizure. Be prepared to assist ventilations if the child experiences benzodiazepine-induced respiratory depression.

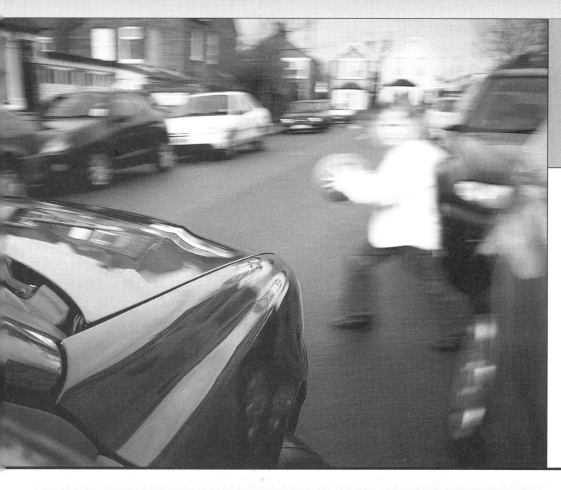

6
6-Year-Old Female Struck by an Automobile

At 1:45 PM on a Saturday afternoon, you are dispatched to the 300 Block of West Highland Street, where a 6-year-old female has been struck by a car. You and your paramedic partner immediately respond to the scene, with a response time of approximately 6 minutes.

Upon arriving at the scene, you find the child lying supine, approximately 15 feet in front of the car that struck her. She appears to be unconscious and is bleeding from the mouth. While your partner stabilizes the child's head and opens her airway with a jaw-thrust maneuver, you perform an initial assessment (**Table 6-1**). Another ambulance with two EMT-Bs arrives to provide assistance.

Table 6-1 Initial Assessment

Level of Consciousness	Responds to painful stimuli; occasional moaning
Mechanism of Injury	Struck by a car
Airway and Breathing	Blood is freely flowing from the mouth; respirations are rapid, gurgling, and irregular.
Circulation	Radial pulse, slow and bounding; skin, warm and dry; blood in the oropharynx; no other gross bleeding

1. What immediate care must you provide to this child?

_____

_____

_____

_____

Your partner and one of the EMT-Bs begin the appropriate management for this child. Further assessment of her mental status reveals a Glasgow Coma Scale of 8 (**Table 6-2**). The driver of the car that struck the child states that she ran out into the street from between two parked cars, and that he was traveling approximately 30 MPH at the time of impact.

Table 6-2 Your Patient's Glasgow Coma Scale

Eye Opening	To pain (2)
Verbal Response	Incomprehensible (2)
Motor Response	Withdraws from pain (4)

2. What is the typical injury pattern when a car strikes a child?

_____

_____

_____

_____

Your partner has cleared the child's airway of blood and prepares to perform endotracheal intubation as the EMT-B continues ventilations. You perform a rapid trauma assessment (**Table 6-3**) as the other EMT-B retrieves a cervical collar, spine board, and straps from the ambulance.

Table 6-3 Rapid Trauma Assessment

Head and Face	Hematoma to the right side of the head, abrasions to the right side of the face, minor oropharyngeal bleeding
Neck	Trachea is midline, jugular veins are normal, no cervical spine deformities.
Chest	Abrasions to left lateral chest; chest wall is stable and symmetrical; breath sounds clear to auscultation bilaterally
Abdomen and Pelvis	Abdomen, soft and nondistended; pelvis, stable to palpation
Extremities (Upper and Lower)	Closed deformity to left femur, abrasions to the left upper extremity
Posterior	No signs of trauma

After administering sedation and a neuromuscular blocking drug (paralytic), your partner has successfully intubated the child and has confirmed correct tube placement by auscultation and capnography. After securing the ET tube, you perform full spinal motion restriction precautions and quickly load the child into the ambulance. Shortly before departing the scene, you obtain baseline vital signs (**Table 6-4**); however, because of the child's decreased level of consciousness and the absence of any relatives, you are unable to obtain a SAMPLE history. You also apply a cardiac monitor.

Table 6-4 Baseline Vital Signs and SAMPLE History

Blood Pressure	140/90 mm Hg
Pulse	66 beats/min, regular and bounding
Respirations	Intubated; ventilated at a rate of 20 breaths/min
Oxygen Saturation	95% (ventilated with 100% oxygen)
Pupils	Bilaterally dilated, sluggishly reactive
ECG	Sinus bradycardia
Signs and Symptoms	Unconscious, head injury, inadequate breathing, extremity trauma
Allergies	Unknown
Medications	Unknown
Pertinent Past History	Unknown
Last Oral Intake	Unknown
Events Leading to Injury	According to the driver, "The child ran out in front of my car, and I couldn't stop in time."

3. What is the pathophysiologic basis for this child's abnormal vital signs?

_____

_____

_____

_____

You ask one of the EMT-Bs to drive the ambulance to a trauma center located 10 miles away. En route, airway management is continued and an IV line of normal saline is established with a large-bore catheter. Dispatch advises you that the police have notified the child's father, who will meet you at the hospital.

4. What is the appropriate prehospital management for this child's condition?

You continue the appropriate treatment for this child's condition, which appears to have improved. Because you will be arriving at the trauma center within the next 5 minutes, you are unable to perform a detailed physical examination. After performing an ongoing assessment (**Table 6-5**), you call your radio report to the receiving facility.

Table 6-5 Ongoing Assessment

Level of Consciousness	Unconscious (sedated and pharmacologically paralyzed)
Airway and Breathing	Intubated; ventilated at a rate of 20 breaths/min
Oxygen Saturation	98% (ventilated with 100% oxygen)
Blood Pressure	130/80 mm Hg
Pulse	88 beats/min, strong and regular
ECG	Normal sinus rhythm

You arrive at the trauma center and are immediately greeted by the attending physician and a trauma surgeon. The child is further stabilized in the emergency department and then taken for a computer tomographic (CT) scan of her abdomen, chest, spine, and head. Following surgical treatment for her injuries, the child is admitted to the pediatric ICU. She recovered with only a mild neurologic deficit.

1. What immediate care must you provide to this child?

This child's airway is in serious jeopardy and requires immediate treatment. Since you have already manually stabilized the child's head and opened her airway with the jaw-thrust maneuver, the following interventions must be performed without delay:

- **Obtain and maintain a patent airway.**
  - This child's airway is at high risk for aspiration; therefore, oropharyngeal suctioning must be performed immediately.
    - Limit suction attempts to 10 seconds at a time.

This child is not completely unconscious and probably has an intact gag reflex; therefore, she is likely to gag if you attempt to insert an oropharyngeal airway. Conversely, because of the potential for significant head trauma, a nasopharyngeal airway should be avoided. In addition, early intubation may be required to maintain airway patency; however, the child must be adequately preoxygenated first.

- **Ventilatory support (bag-valve-mask device)**
  - Ventilate the child at a rate of 20 breaths/min.
    - Respirations that are too rapid or too slow, shallow, and irregular will not produce the amount of tidal volume (and thus minute volume) needed to support life.
    - Passive oxygenation with a nonrebreathing mask is **only** effective if the child is breathing adequately (eg, adequate rate and tidal volume) and is able to inhale the oxygen without assistance.
    - A nonrebreathing mask will **not** provide positive-pressure ventilation, which is needed in this child to restore adequate tidal volume.

The priorities of airway management are no different in the child than they are in the adult—open, clear, assess, and manage. Although this child will require intubation for definitive airway control, her airway must be managed by utilizing basic means first. Avoid the temptation to proceed with immediate advanced airway management, unless the child's airway cannot be controlled by any other means.

Before respiratory effort can be assessed and managed, the airway must be clear of obstructions such as blood, vomitus, or broken teeth. This child has two major airway problems—oropharyngeal bleeding **and** inadequate breathing, both of which will result in profound hypoxia and death if not treated immediately. The most effective way to manage this child's airway initially is to suction her oropharynx for 10 seconds and then provide positive-pressure ventilations for 2 minutes. This alternating pattern should be continued until the child's airway is clear of blood or she has been intubated. Regardless of the patient's condition, the airway must remain patent at all times.

2. What is the typical injury pattern when a car strikes a child?

During a motor vehicle versus pedestrian collision, children often sustain multiple-systems trauma, especially if the vehicle is traveling at a moderate to high rate of speed. However, the injury pattern that occurs as the result of this type of mechanism of injury is often predictable.

Adult pedestrians typically turn away from the oncoming vehicle before being struck, whereas children commonly turn toward the oncoming vehicle. Upon initial impact, adults are typically thrown onto the hood or into the windshield of the vehicle, whereas children, because of their smaller size, tend to be thrown in front of the vehicle.

Initial impact occurs when the vehicle's bumper strikes the child's abdomen, pelvis, or femur; the exact area of impact depends on the child's height and the height of the vehicle's bumper at the time of impact. The initial impact results in blunt abdominal trauma, pelvic fractures, or femur fractures. Blunt thoracic trauma occurs during the second impact, when the child's chest strikes the vehicle's grille or hood. Closed head trauma occurs when the child is propelled away from the vehicle and strikes his or her head on the ground (**Figure 6-1**). This relatively predictable injury pattern is referred to as Waddell's triad (**Table 6-6**).

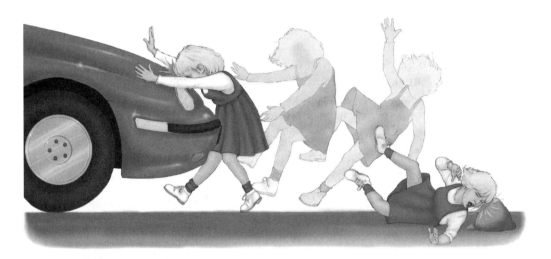

■ **Figure 6-1** Waddell's triad is a predictable injury pattern commonly seen when an automobile strikes a child.

Table 6-6 Waddell's Triad

Initial impact
- Blunt abdominal trauma, pelvic fractures, and/or femur injuries
  - Occurs when the child is struck by the bumper
  - Exact area of impact depends on the child's height and the height of the vehicle's bumper at the time of impact.

Second impact
- Thoracic trauma
  - Occurs when the child strikes the grille or hood of the vehicle

Third impact
- Closed head trauma
  - Occurs when the child is propelled away from the vehicle and strikes his or her head on the ground

Of these three injury patterns, traumatic brain injury (TBI) is associated with the highest mortality rate when a car strikes a child. Therefore, early and aggressive airway management, with simultaneous cervical spine control, is critical to the child's survival.

The ribs are very pliable in a child and offer little protection for the internal thoracic organs (**Figure 6-2**). Because signs of external trauma are often minimal or absent, life-threatening intrathoracic injuries in the child may be overlooked if a careful, systematic assessment is not performed.

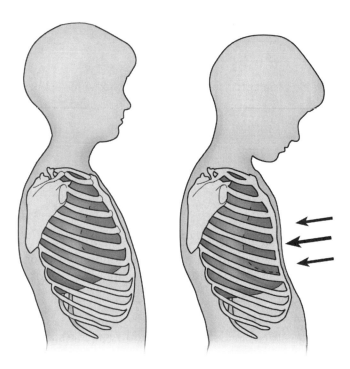

■ **Figure 6-2** A child's ribs are more pliable than an adult's. As a result, life-threatening intrathoracic trauma can occur with little or no external signs of injury.

Unless associated with internal bleeding, lower extremities fractures are usually not life-threatening. If not properly managed, however, long-term complications, such as abnormal bone development, can occur.

3. What is the pathophysiologic basis for this child's abnormal vital signs?

This child is experiencing increased intracranial pressure (ICP) as the result of closed head trauma and cerebral edema. Her abnormal vital signs, albeit ominous, follow a rather predictable pattern.

Hypertension is common in patients with increased ICP, and is the result of the body's attempt to maintain cerebral blood flow and cerebral perfusion pressure (CPP) by shunting more blood to the injured brain—a process called autoregulation (also called Cushing's reflex).

Because of the acute rise in systolic BP, a reflex bradycardia occurs as a result of increased parasympathetic tone. Small children who are unconscious, apneic (or breathing inadequately), and who are displaying signs of poor perfusion should receive chest compressions (rate of 100 compressions/min) if their heart rate falls below 60 beats per minute.

As ICP continues to rise, pressure is placed on various levels of the brain stem, which results in a variety of abnormal respiratory patterns. Such patterns include central neurogenic hyperventilation, Cheyne-Stokes respirations, and ataxic (Biot's) respirations. These respiratory patterns usually produce inadequate tidal volume and will require ventilatory support.

This trio of abnormal vital signs—hypertension, bradycardia, and abnormal breathing—is referred to as "Cushing's triad" (**Table 6-7**) and is a classic finding associated with increased ICP.

Table 6-7 Cushing's Triad

Hypertension
- The result of systemic vasoconstriction in order to shunt more blood to the injured brain (autoregulation [Cushing's reflex])

Bradycardia
- Reflex response to an acute rise in systolic BP, caused by increased parasympathetic tone

Abnormal respirations
- Caused by pressure on various levels of the brain stem

4. What is the appropriate prehospital management for this child's condition?

In addition to maintaining airway patency and applying full spinal motion restriction precautions, the Brain Trauma Foundation (BTF) recommends the following prehospital treatment guidelines for the brain-injured child:

■ **Ensure adequate oxygenation and ventilation.**
- Continue ventilatory assistance because this child's rapid and irregular respirations are not producing adequate tidal volume.
- In the child, provide ventilations at a rate of 20 breaths per minute.
  - Hyperventilate at a rate of 30 breaths/min *only* if signs of brain herniation are present.

Routine hyperventilation should be avoided in the brain-injured patient with elevated ICP, unless signs of brain herniation are present (**Table 6-8**). Hyperventilation causes a rapid decrease in the partial pressure of carbon dioxide in arterial blood ($PaCO_2$), which causes cerebral vasoconstriction and decreased cerebral blood flow. Although cerebral vasoconstriction will shunt blood from the brain and lower ICP, it will only give the brain more room to swell within the cranial vault.

Table 6-8 Signs of Brain Herniation

An unresponsive (comatose) patient with *both* of the following:
- Bilaterally dilated and unresponsive pupils *or* unequal pupils
- Decerebrate (extensor) posturing *or* no motor response to painful stimuli

Herniation, which occurs when the brain itself is forced from the cranial vault through the foramen magnum (opening at the base of the skull), indicates markedly elevated ICP. Clinically, herniation manifests with ominous signs, such as unilaterally or bilaterally dilated and unresponsive pupils and decorticate (flexor) or decerebrate (extensor) posturing (**Figure 6-3**).

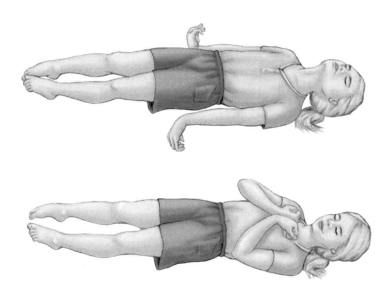

■ **Figure 6-3** Decerebrate posturing (top) and decorticate posturing (bottom) are ominous signs of increased ICP and indicate brain herniation.

After adequately preoxygenating the child, endotracheal intubation should be performed to definitively secure and protect her airway. Many patients with closed head trauma and ICP are combative and/or have clenched teeth (trismus); therefore, pharmacological agents (eg, sedation, neuromuscular blockers [paralytics]) may be required in order to facilitate intubation. Be sure to adequately secure the ET tube and frequently reassess tube placement through auscultation and capnography.

Digital capnometry, if available, should be used in conjunction with intubation. Digital capnometry allows for continuous assessment of ET tube placement by providing data that is continuous, quantitative, and in real time. In addition, you can approximate the patient's $PaCO_2$, which, in the brain-injured patient, should be maintained between 30 and 35 mm Hg.

Continuously monitor and maintain the child's oxygen saturation (SaO_2) at 90% or higher (clearly, the higher the better). A *single* drop in SaO_2 to less than 90% doubles the brain-injured patient's chances of death.

■ **Maintain systolic blood pressure.**
  • At present, this child is hypertensive (140/90 mm Hg); therefore, set your IV line(s) to run at a keep-vein-open rate.
  • Be prepared to infuse isotonic crystalloids (eg, normal saline, lactated Ringer's solution) to maintain perfusion if hypotension occurs.

Hypotension in a child between 6 and 12 years of age exists when the systolic BP falls below 80 mm Hg. Hypotension in the brain-injured patient can have disastrous consequences; it causes diminished cerebral blood flow and impairs cerebral perfusion pressure (CPP).

CPP must remain adequate in order to maintain sufficient cerebral blood flow. A CPP of less than 60 mm Hg (critical minimum threshold) will result in cerebral ischemia, clearly increasing mortality from traumatic brain injury.

CPP is computed by subtracting the patient's intracranial pressure, the upper limit of normal being 15 mm Hg, from the mean arterial pressure (MAP). MAP is calculated by using the following formula:

$$\text{MAP} = \text{systolic BP} + \text{diastolic BP} \ (\times \ 2) \div 3$$

Although ICP cannot be measured in the field, let's assume that in this particular child, it is 20 mm Hg (it should be no greater than 15 mm Hg). To demonstrate the deleterious effects of hypotension, we will calculate her CPP, using both her initial blood pressure reading of 140/90 mm Hg and a hypotensive blood pressure of 70/40 mm Hg.

Example 1: CPP based on a blood pressure of 140/90 mm Hg
- 140 (SBP) + 180 (DBP × 2) = 320 ÷ 3 = 107 (MAP)
- 107 (MAP) − 20 (ICP) = *87 (CPP)*

Example 2: CPP based on a blood pressure of 70/40 mm Hg:
- 70 (SBP) + 80 (DBP × 2) = 150 ÷ 3 = 50 (MAP)
- 50 (MAP) − 20 (ICP) = *30 (CPP)*

From the above examples, it is clear that maintaining the brain-injured patient's blood pressure is critical to his or her survival. IV crystalloid boluses of 20 mL/kg should be infused to maintain a systolic BP of at least 80 mm Hg in the child. A *single* drop in systolic BP to less than 80 mm Hg in the brain-injured child doubles his or her chances of death.

The ultimate goal of intravenous therapy in the brain-injured patient is to maintain cerebral perfusion pressure *without* exacerbating intracranial pressure. Since this can be a fine balance to maintain, your intravenous line(s) must be titrated carefully, while constantly monitoring the patient. In the absence of hypotension, IV fluids should be restricted in the brain-injured patient to minimize cerebral edema and ICP.

The Glasgow Coma Scale (GCS) is a valuable assessment tool, and is the most widely employed method for reporting serial neurological evaluations. The GCS is the same for the child as it is for the adult; however, the infant GCS is different in order to accommodate their age-specific behavior (eg, cooing, babbling).

Deterioration of the patient's GCS by 2 or more points, **or** a *single* drop in the GCS below 9, doubles the brain-injured patient's chances of death. A GCS of 14 to 15 indicates mild brain injury; a GCS of 9 to 13 indicates moderate brain injury; and a GCS of 3 to 8 indicates severe brain injury. Remember, however, that these are merely numbers; you must relay the specific area(s) of the GCS that are abnormal.

Because a single GCS measurement cannot possibly predict the brain-injured patient's outcome, it should be reassessed at least every 5 minutes. Maintain documentation of the patient's GCS recordings and report them to the emergency department physician.

Pharmacological therapy, other than that required to facilitate intubation or treat seizures, is generally not indicated in the prehospital setting for the brain-injured patient. Follow locally established protocols regarding which, if any, medications are to be used in the brain-injured patient.

As with any critically injured patient, rapid transport to a trauma center is essential in the overall management of the brain-injured patient. Notify the receiving facility early, so that the appropriate resources (eg, CT scan, surgery) can be allocated.

Summary

According to the Brain Trauma Foundation, brain injury is the leading cause of traumatic death in children, accounting for 30% to 50% of all pediatric trauma deaths. Pedestrian accidents account for approximately 20% of all cases of pediatric head trauma.

Death from serious brain injury is usually the result of cerebral edema, increased ICP, and anoxic brain injury; this is often complicated by the presence of a spinal injury. If not promptly treated, the traumatized brain will continue to swell, and herniation will occur.

Prehospital management for the child with a severe head injury and increased ICP includes maintaining a patent airway, ensuring effective ventilation, applying full spinal motion restriction precautions, and maintaining a systolic BP of at least 80 mm Hg with isotonic crystalloid fluids. Hyperventilation should be avoided unless the child is displaying signs of brain herniation; in such cases, brief periods of hyperventilation may be beneficial. Rapid transport to and early notification of a trauma center are critical, and will significantly increase the child's chances of survival.

Fortunately, children have a better survival rate from serious head trauma than adults, with death occurring only half as often. This is likely due to their cartilaginous skulls and the presence of incompletely fused cranial sutures. These anatomic features allow the skull to stretch somewhat, providing for greater expansion of the brain before it begins to herniate. Nonetheless, the child's skull has its limits; therefore, prompt recognition and treatment of head trauma with elevated ICP and rapid transport are just as critical in the child as they are in the adult.

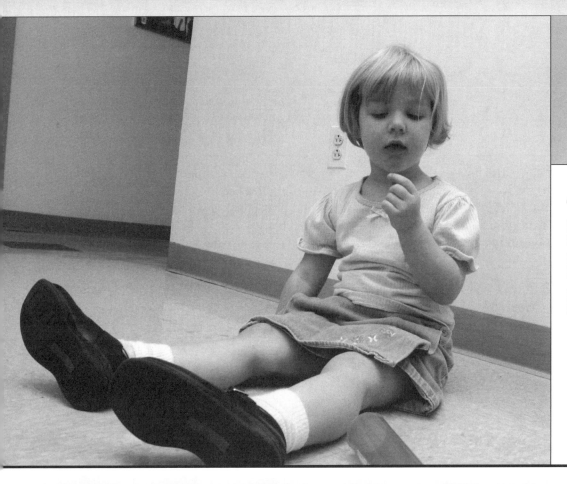

7

4-Year-Old Female Who Ingested a Medication

At 10:45 AM, your unit is dispatched to 565 East Lohman Street for a 4-year-old female who has ingested an unknown medication. While en route to the scene, dispatch advises you that the child is unconscious. Your response time to the scene is approximately 5 minutes.

When you arrive at the scene and enter the residence, you find a woman, who identifies herself as the child's mother, frantically trying to awaken the unconscious child. She tells you that her daughter swallowed an unknown number of her husband's blood pressure pills. You perform an initial assessment (**Table 7-1**) as your partner opens the airway bag.

Table 7-1 Initial Assessment

Level of Consciousness	Unconscious and unresponsive
Chief Complaint	According to the mother, "She took some of my husband's high blood pressure pills. I don't know how many she took."
Airway and Breathing	Airway is patent; respirations, rapid rate and shallow depth
Circulation	Radial pulse, slow and weak; skin, cool and cyanotic; no gross bleeding; capillary refill time, 3 seconds

1. What is the appropriate initial management of this child?

_____

_____

_____

_____

Your partner states that he is meeting resistance while ventilating the child with the bag-valve-mask device, even after repositioning her head to ensure a neutral position. You quickly auscultate the child's lungs and hear bilateral wheezing. The mother hands you an opened bottle of medication labeled "Sectral SR." You look the medication up in your field guide and determine that it is a sustained-release beta-blocker.

2. Why is your partner having difficulty ventilating this child? How should this be treated?

_____

_____

_____

Following the appropriate therapy, your partner is able to provide adequate tidal volume with the bag-valve-mask device. You reauscultate the child's lungs and note scattered wheezing, but to a much lesser degree. You perform a rapid assessment of the child (**Table 7-2**) as your partner continues ventilatory assistance. A police officer arrives at the scene and obtains information from the mother regarding the event.

Table 7-2 Rapid Assessment

Head	No obvious trauma
Neck	Jugular veins are normal; trachea is midline; no cervical spine deformities.
Chest	No obvious trauma, chest movement is symmetrical, scattered wheezing bilaterally
Abdomen	Soft, nondistended, no obvious trauma
Pelvis	Stable to palpation
Extremities (Upper and Lower)	No obvious trauma, distal pulses are weakly palpable.
Posterior	No obvious trauma

After applying a cardiac monitor and assessing the child's cardiac rhythm (**Figure 7-1**), you obtain a blood glucose reading, which is 40 mg/dL. The child's mother states that her daughter is not a diabetic. As you establish an IV of normal saline in preparation for further treatment, the police officer retrieves the stretcher from the ambulance.

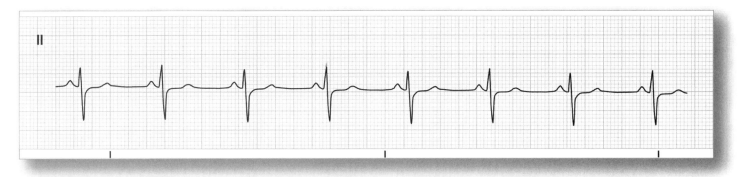

■ **Figure 7-1** The child's cardiac rhythm.

3. What is the etiology of this child's hypoglycemia?

You quickly place the child onto the stretcher and load her into the ambulance. Shortly before departing the scene, you obtain baseline vital signs and a SAMPLE history (**Table 7-3**). The mother, who is sitting in the passenger seat of the ambulance, provides you with her daughter's medical history.

Table 7-3 Baseline Vital Signs and SAMPLE History

Blood Pressure	70/40 mm Hg
Pulse	66 beats/min, weak and regular
Capillary Refill Time	3 seconds
Respirations	48 breaths/min and shallow (baseline); ventilations are being assisted with a bag-valve-mask device and 100% oxygen
Oxygen Saturation	97% (ventilated with 100% oxygen)
Signs and Symptoms	Unresponsive, inadequate breathing, bradycardia, hypotension, hypoglycemia
Allergies	None
Medications	None
Pertinent Past History	None
Child's Weight	According to mother, about 35 pounds (16 kg)
Events Leading to Present Illness	"I guess she got into the medicine cabinet while I wasn't looking. I found her unconscious in her bedroom."

4. What specific treatment is required to treat this child's condition?

_____

_____

_____

Because your partner's assistance is needed in the back with the child, the police officer agrees to drive the ambulance to a pediatric hospital, which is located 15 miles away. En route, you provide the appropriate treatment for the child's condition, while closely monitoring her cardiac rhythm.

5. What additional cardiac problems can beta-blocker toxicity cause?

_____

_____

_____

Following the appropriate treatment, you begin to notice improvement in the child's condition. Her level of consciousness is improving and she is now resisting ventilatory support. Your partner applies a nonrebreathing mask at 15 L/min and closely monitors her oxygen saturation. You reassess the child's cardiac rhythm, and note that it has improved (**Figure 7-2**).

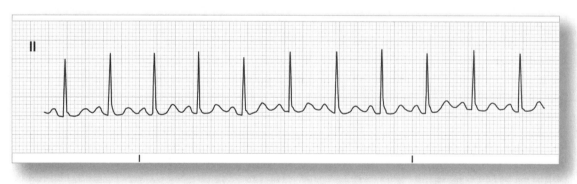

■ **Figure 7-2** The child's cardiac rhythm has improved.

You reassess the child's blood glucose level, which reads 102 mg/dL. With an estimated time of arrival at the hospital of 7 minutes, you perform an ongoing assessment (**Table 7-4**) and then call your radio report to the receiving facility.

Table 7-4 Ongoing Assessment

Level of Consciousness	Appears sleepy, crying
Airway and Breathing	Airway remains patent; respirations, 30 breaths/min; adequate tidal volume
Oxygen Saturation	98% (on 100% oxygen)
Blood Pressure	80/50 mm Hg
Pulse	120 beats/min, strong and regular
Capillary Refill Time	1-2 seconds
Blood Glucose	102 mg/dL
ECG	Normal sinus rhythm

6. How can sustained-release (SR) medications affect this child's condition?

_____

_____

_____

_____

You deliver the child to the emergency department in stable condition and give your verbal report to the attending physician. After additional assessment and management in the emergency department, the child is admitted to the pediatric ICU for observation. She later recovered and was discharged home.

1. What is the appropriate initial management of this child?

■ Obtain and maintain a patent airway.
- After opening the child's airway with the appropriate maneuver, an airway adjunct should be inserted to maintain a patent airway.
  - In the unconscious patient, an oropharyngeal airway should be inserted unless a gag reflex is present.
  - If the child will not tolerate an oropharyngeal airway, insert a nasopharyngeal airway.
- Be prepared to suction the child's airway if vomiting occurs.

■ Ventilatory support
- This child's respiratory effort is producing inadequate tidal volume, as evidenced by the minimal rise of her chest.
- Assist ventilations with a pediatric-sized bag-valve-mask device or pocket-mask device.

Rapid or slow respirations, especially with shallow depth (reduced tidal volume), will not result in sufficient minute volume to support life. Because the oxygen delivered by a nonrebreathing mask will not effectively be drawn into the lungs of a patient with inadequate breathing, positive-pressure ventilatory support is needed.

Another indication of the need for positive-pressure ventilations in the child is bradycardia, especially if accompanied by an altered mental status and signs of poor perfusion (eg, cyanosis, pallor).

Although this child's bradycardia is likely due to the ingestion of a medication that will require specific therapy, the initial management is no different than that of any other child (or patient, for that matter) with inadequate respiratory effort—ventilatory and oxygenation support!

2. Why is your partner having difficulty ventilating this child? How should this be treated?

Decreased ventilatory compliance (increased ventilatory difficulty) is commonly the result of inadequate positioning of the child's head. Proportionately, children have larger heads than adults, specifically the occipital region of the skull. If the head is not placed in a neutral position, the large occiput can push the entire head forward, causing obstruction of the airway. To correct this, place padding underneath the child's shoulders to maintain a neutral head position.

Decreased ventilatory compliance in this child is the result of severe bronchospasm, as evidenced by the diffuse wheezing. Bronchospasm is a common finding in cases of beta-blocker toxicity.

Beta-adrenergic blockers, such as acebutolol (Sectral), propranolol (Inderal), and metoprolol (Lopressor), compete with epinephrine and norepinephrine—the neurotransmitters of the sympathetic nervous system—at the beta-adrenergic receptors. Beta-adrenergic receptors are divided into two subtypes—beta$_1$ and beta$_2$. Beta$_1$ receptors are located primarily in cardiac and renal tissue, and beta$_2$ receptors are located in the liver and smooth muscle of the blood vessels, trachea, bronchi, and gastrointestinal tract.

When beta$_2$ receptors are excessively blocked, as seen with beta-blocker overdose, the result is severe bronchospasm, which results in increased airway resistance. Although this is especially common in children with preexisting reactive airway diseases (eg, asthma), it can occur in anyone with beta-blocker toxicity. Severe bronchospasm, and the resultant increased airway resistance that it causes, make adequate tidal volume difficult to achieve when providing positive-pressure ventilations.

The treatment is therefore aimed at agonizing (stimulating) beta$_2$ receptors sites, which is most effectively accomplished by administering a nebulized bronchodilator, such as albuterol (Ventolin, Proventil), metaproterenol (Alupent), or isoetharine (Bronkosol). These drugs selectively target beta$_2$ receptors sites, causing relaxation of bronchiole smooth muscle, and thus, bronchodilation.

When using a bag-valve-mask device, bronchodilators can be administered via a small-volume inline nebulizer. This allows you to provide positive-pressure ventilations to maintain adequate tidal volume, while treating the bronchospasm at the same time. Continuous bronchodilator therapy is often required in cases of severe bronchospasm.

Albuterol is the most commonly administered nebulized bronchodilator, because of its high margin of safety. The pediatric dose of albuterol depends on the child's weight:

- < 15 kg (< 33 lb): 2.5–5 mg (0.5–1 mL) diluted in 3 mL of normal saline
- > 15 kg (> 33 lb): 5–10 mg (1–2 mL) diluted in 3 mL of normal saline

3. What is the etiology of this child's hypoglycemia?

As previously discussed, beta$_2$ receptors are located in the liver, which, when stimulated by catecholamines, result in two biochemical processes that increase the body's supply of blood sugar—glycogenolysis and gluconeogenesis. These biochemical processes are regulated by glucagon, a hormonal protein produced in the alpha cells of the pancreas.

During glycogenolysis, glucagon stimulates the liver to convert glycogen (a complex sugar) to glucose (a simpler sugar), which is converted to energy by the body. Gluconeogenesis occurs when glucagon stimulates the production of new (nonglycogen) glucose from the breakdown of fats and fatty acids.

When beta$_2$ receptors are blocked, these biochemical processes that maintain adequate blood glucose levels are blocked as well. As a result, blood glucose can fall to dangerously low levels (hypoglycemia).

Hypoglycemia caused by beta-blocker toxicity is especially common in children, who already have limited stores of glycogen in their liver. During shock caused by beta-blocker toxicity, which is usually secondary to bradycardia and hypotension, the child will rapidly deplete what little sugar he or she has in an attempt to compensate for the low cardiac output state. Blood glucose levels lower than 60 mg/dL often cause or contribute to altered mental status.

It is important for the paramedic to perform a careful and systematic assessment of the child who has ingested a beta-blocker, including routine blood glucose testing. Hypoglycemia, which is easily treated, will cause permanent brain damage or even death of the patient if it is not quickly identified or is left untreated.

4. What specific treatment is required to treat this child's condition?

Excessive beta$_1$ receptor blockade decreases heart rate (chronotropy), electrical conduction velocity (dromotropy), and myocardial contractility (inotropy), resulting in bradycardia, hypotension, and systemic hypoperfusion (shock). Additionally, beta$_2$ receptor blockade often causes hypoglycemia; which, as previously discussed, is especially common in children.

After ensuring adequate oxygenation and ventilation and establishing vascular access, specific treatment for this child should focus on treating hypoglycemia and increasing heart rate and blood pressure. The American Academy of Pediatrics (AAP) recommends the following treatment for pediatric beta-blocker toxicity:

- **Glucagon 0.05 to 0.1 mg/kg via IV administration (up to 1 mg)**
  - Glucagon is used for beta-blocker toxicity primarily because of its positive chronotropic and inotropic effects, which are unrelated to beta$_1$ receptor stimulation.
    - Glucagon is effective in increasing heart rate and blood pressure associated with beta-blocker toxicity.
  - If IV access is not available, administer 1 mg glucagon via IM injection.
    - Repeat at 1 mg in 20 minutes as needed.

Glucagon may also be effective in restoring adequate blood glucose levels by facilitating the processes of glycogenolysis and gluconeogenesis. However, glucagon will only be effective if there are adequate stores of glycogen in the liver, which is not always the case in children. If glucagon administration is not allowed by locally established protocols and the child's blood glucose level is less than 60 mg/dL, administer 0.5 to 1 g/kg of 25% dextrose (D_{25}) via IV or IO administration.

A catecholamine infusion should be considered to treat bradycardia and hypotension if glucagon is not effective or not allowed by locally established protocols. Although dopamine (Intropin) and norepinephrine (Levophed) can be used, epinephrine (Adrenalin) often produces better results, especially when the hypotension is associated with bradycardia. The pediatric infusion dose of epinephrine is as follows:

- **0.1 to 1 µg/kg/min**
  - Increase the infusion as needed to increase heart rate and blood pressure.
  - High infusion doses are often needed to overcome significant beta blockade.

If the child is unresponsive to glucagon and epinephrine, transcutaneous cardiac pacing may be indicated to treat the bradycardia. Refer to locally established protocols or contact medical control as needed regarding additional pharmacological management of beta-blocker toxicity.

5. What additional cardiac problems can beta-blocker toxicity cause?

In addition to causing bradycardia, beta-blocker toxicity can also result in PR interval prolongation, various degrees of AV heart block, intraventricular conduction delays, and widening of the QRS and QT intervals.

Acebutolol (Sectral) is one of the most toxic beta-blockers when taken excessively, and, unlike other beta-blockers (eg, Inderal), may predispose the patient to ventricular repolarization abnormalities. Therefore, the patient could experience lethal ventricular arrhythmias, such as V-tach (with or without a pulse) or V-fib. It is therefore important to continuously monitor the child's cardiac rhythm, even after symptoms begin to resolve. If V-fib or pulseless V-tach occurs, perform immediate defibrillation. **Table 7-5** summarizes the signs and symptoms, by body system, of beta-blocker toxicity.

Table 7-5 Signs and Symptoms of Beta-Blocker Toxicity

Central nervous system
- Altered mental status
- Seizures

Cardiovascular
- Bradycardia
- Hypotension
- Prolongation of the QRS, PR, and QT intervals
- Various degrees of AV heart block
- Ventricular arrhythmias

Respiratory
- Bronchospasm
- Increased airway resistance

Metabolic
- Hypoglycemia

6. How can sustained-release (SR) medications affect this child's condition?

Sustained-release (SR) medications are prescribed in order to maintain a longer therapeutic effect, thus requiring minimal dosing. Because this child has ingested a sustained-release form of the beta-blocker, her symptoms may be prolonged, or may recur following treatment. Therefore, continuous monitoring of her condition, including the ABCs, blood pressure, and cardiac rhythm, is essential.

During your radio report to the receiving facility, you must inform them of the type of medication ingested, including whether or not the medication is a sustained-release form, the estimated amount of the ingestion, the approximate time in which the ingestion occurred, and whether or not any home remedies were provided. This will allow the attending physician to direct his or her treatment accordingly.

Summary

Beta-blockers are widely prescribed for a number of medical conditions, such as hypertension and supraventricular tachycardia (SVT). They are also responsible for a large number of accidental ingestions, especially in children.

Beta-blockers compete with epinephrine and norepinephrine (catecholamines) at the beta-adrenergic receptors, which are located in the heart, kidneys, liver, and the smooth muscles of the blood vessels, trachea, and gastrointestinal tract.

Clinical signs of beta-blocker toxicity include bradycardia, hypotension, bronchospasm, and hypoglycemia (especially in children). Mental status is commonly altered and may be complicated by hypoxia- or hypoglycemia-induced seizures.

The initial management for the child with beta-blocker toxicity includes supporting airway, breathing, and circulation. Nebulized bronchodilators (eg, albuterol, Alupent) may be needed to relieve bronchospasm and facilitate assisted ventilations. Monitor the child's cardiac rhythm for AV heart blocks, QRS widening, and ventricular arrhythmias.

Pharmacological management for beta-blocker toxicity includes glucagon, which is used for its positive inotropic and chronotropic effects. Glucagon may also be useful in restoring adequate blood glucose levels. For glucagon-refractory hypoglycemia, D_{25} should be administered.

Catecholamine infusions, epinephrine being the most common, should be administered if glucagon fails to increase the patient's heart rate and blood pressure. However, higher-than-normal infusion doses may be needed. Refer to locally established protocols or contact medical control regarding additional pharmacological management of beta-blocker toxicity.

Sustained-release (SR) beta-blockers may cause prolonged symptoms, or the recurrence of original symptoms following treatment. Therefore, continuous monitoring of the patient is essential.

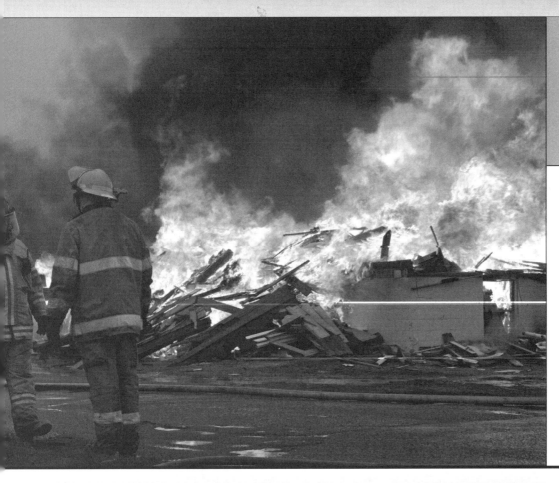

8

9-Year-Old Male with Severe Burns

At 5:30 PM, the fire department requests your assistance at the scene of a structural fire involving a local restaurant, where they have rescued a 9-year-old male from the burning building. Apparently, the child was trapped in the building's bathroom at the time of the fire. You immediately proceed to the scene, with a response time of approximately 5 minutes.

You arrive at the scene at 5:35 PM. Fire fighters have stopped the burning process, covered the child with a blanket, placed him in a supine position, and have applied 100% oxygen via nonrebreathing mask. You remove the blanket to quickly assess the child's burns, and note that he has partial- and full-thickness burns to his head, face, trunk, and upper extremities. Your partner maintains manual stabilization of the child's head as you perform an initial assessment (Table 8-1).

Table 8-1 Initial Assessment

Level of Consciousness	Responsive to painful stimuli only
Mechanism of Injury	Trapped in a burning building; possible toxic exposure
Airway and Breathing	Carbonaceous sputum in the mouth and nose; singed nasal hair; respirations are rapid and shallow.
Circulation	Radial pulse, rapid and thready; skin, cool and pale; capillary refill time, 4 seconds; no gross bleeding

1. How should you manage this child's airway initially?

With a fire fighter's assistance, your partner initiates the appropriate airway management for the child. After performing a rapid trauma assessment (**Table 8-2**), you place a sterile burn sheet and blanket on the child, perform full spinal motion restriction precautions, and quickly load him into the ambulance.

Table 8-2 Rapid Trauma Assessment

Head	Partial- and full-thickness burns to the head and face, no deformities or bleeding
Neck	Partial-thickness burns to the anterior neck; jugular veins, flat; trachea, midline
Chest	Partial- and full-thickness burns to the anterior chest; breath sounds, distant but equal bilaterally; chest wall is stable and symmetrical
Abdomen	Partial- and full-thickness burns to the abdomen; abdomen is soft and non-tender
Pelvis	Stable to palpation
Extremities (Upper and Lower)	Partial- and full-thickness burns to both anterior upper extremities; no obvious trauma to the lower extremities; distal pulses, weakly present
Posterior	No obvious trauma

2. What percentage of this child's body surface area has been burned?

_____

_____

_____

The child's respirations are becoming markedly stridorous and labored, and his oxygen saturation reads 88%. Your partner states that ventilations are becoming increasingly difficult to perform. After placing an intraosseous (IO) catheter in the child's proximal tibia, you assist your partner with the child's airway.

3. How should you manage this child's airway now?

_____

_____

_____

The child's airway has been definitively secured and ventilatory assistance is continued at the appropriate rate. Because your partner's assistance is needed in the back with the patient, you ask a fire fighter to drive the ambulance to a trauma center, which is located 15 miles away. Shortly before departing the scene, you obtain baseline vital signs and a SAMPLE history (**Table 8-3**).

Table 8-3 Baseline Vital Signs and SAMPLE History

Blood Pressure	Unable to obtain (burned upper extremities)
Pulse	150 beats/min, regular and weak
Respirations	Intubated; ventilations are being assisted.
Capillary Refill Time	4 seconds
Oxygen Saturation	95% (intubated and ventilated)
Blood Glucose	98 mg/dL
Signs and Symptoms	Severe burns to the head, face, torso, and upper extremities
Allergies	Unknown
Medications	Unknown
Pertinent Past History	Unknown
Last Oral Intake	Unknown
Events Leading to Injury	Trapped in a burning building for an unknown period of time

4. Why are burns more life-threatening in children than in adults?

_____

_____

_____

_____

En route to the trauma center, you insert a second IO catheter in the child and begin the appropriate fluid resuscitation. A cardiac monitor is applied and reveals a sinus tachycardia at 150 beats/min. As your partner continues ventilatory assistance, you note that the child's oxygen saturation has increased to 97%.

5. What is the appropriate IV fluid therapy for this child?

_____

_____

_____

_____

Following aggressive treatment en route to the trauma center, you note improvement in the child's condition. His capillary refill time is 2 to 3 seconds and his heart rate is now 120 beats/min. Without time to perform a detailed physical examination, you perform an ongoing assessment (**Table 8-4**) of the child, and then call your radio report to the receiving facility.

Table 8-4 Ongoing Assessment

Level of Consciousness	Sedated and intubated
Airway and Breathing	Intubated, ventilations are being assisted
Oxygen Saturation	97% (intubated and ventilated)
Blood Pressure	Not obtained (burned upper extremities)
Pulse	120 beats/min, stronger and regular
Capillary Refill Time	2 to 3 seconds
Blood Glucose	100 mg/dL

The child is delivered to the trauma center, where a team of physicians is awaiting your arrival. Following additional assessment and treatment in the emergency department, the child was treated with hyperbaric therapy for significant carbon monoxide (CO) toxicity. Following resolution of his CO toxicity, the child was transferred by air to a burn center for specific burn management. He later recovered and was transferred to a rehabilitation facility.

8

1. How should you manage this child's airway initially?

■ **Oropharyngeal suctioning**

Secretions in the airway pose a risk for aspiration and severe hypoxia, and should thus be removed with suction. In children, oropharyngeal suctioning should be limited to 10 seconds per attempt. Avoid vigorous suctioning, since this may exacerbate soft-tissue swelling if the child has experienced upper airway burns.

■ **Airway adjunct**

Consider inserting a nasopharyngeal airway to help maintain patency of the child's airway. Although his level of consciousness is markedly diminished (responsive to pain only), he will likely gag if you attempt to insert an oropharyngeal airway.

■ **Positive-pressure ventilatory assistance**

This child's decreased level of consciousness is likely due to hypoxia, CO toxicity, or both. Cyanide, also a common byproduct found in structural fires, should be considered as well. Rapid respirations with shallow depth are not producing the amount of tidal volume (and minute volume) needed to support life. Therefore, positive-pressure ventilatory assistance with a bag-valve-mask device and 100% oxygen is indicated.

A nonrebreathing mask, because it will not deliver oxygen via positive-pressure, is of minimal to no value to the inadequately breathing patient. Sufficient intake of passive oxygenation with a nonrebreathing mask is dependant upon adequate ventilation (eg, adequate rate and tidal volume).

Because of the singed nasal hair and carbonaceous sputum in the child's nose and mouth, you must closely monitor his airway for signs of swelling that would necessitate early intubation. Such signs include, among others, stridor and increasing dyspnea.

2. What percentage of this child's body surface area has been burned?

This child has experienced partial- and full-thickness burns that cover approximately 39% of his body surface area (BSA) (**Table 8-5**). Because children have proportionately larger body surface areas, modified burn assessment charts are necessary in order to accurately determine the extent of their BSA burns (**Figure 8-1**).

Table 8-5 Your Patient's BSA Extent of Burn

Head and neck: 12%
Anterior chest and abdomen: 18%
Bilateral anterior upper extremities: 9% • Each *complete* upper extremity is equal to 9% of the child's BSA.

Although estimating the extent of the child's BSA that has been burned is important, it is of equal if not of more importance to determine the degree (depth) and the anatomic location of the burns. This is especially important when calling your radio report to the receiving facility. Simply stating that the child has sustained burns to 39% of his BSA does not provide an accurate description of the child's condition. As a result, the physician will not know what kind of injuries to expect when he or she receives the patient. Instead, advise the receiving facility that the child has sustained partial- and full- thickness burns to 39% of his BSA, and then state the exact location of the burns.

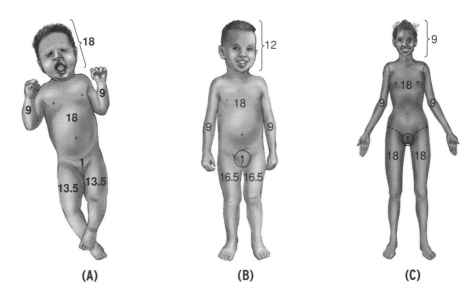

■ **Figure 8-1** A modified anatomic map of children of different ages gives an approximation of involved body surface area for calculation of burn extent in (A) infant, (B) child, and (C) adolescent.

Another quick method for calculating the extent of the BSA burned is the "rule of palms" (**Figure 8-2**), which states that the patient's hand (minus the fingers) is equal to 1% of their total BSA. The percent of burned BSA is therefore roughly equal to the number of patient palm-sized areas burned.

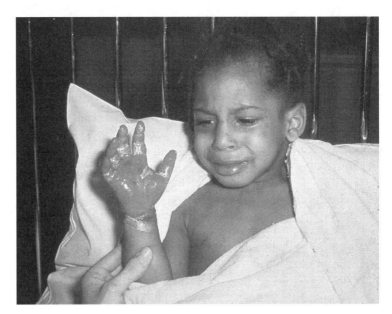

■ **Figure 8-2** The palm is approximately 1% of the body surface area.

3. How should you manage this child's airway now?

■ Endotracheal intubation

As evidenced by his markedly stridorous and labored respirations, distant breath sounds during auscultation, and falling oxygen saturation (SaO_2), this child is experiencing upper airway swelling, increasing hypoxia, and impending airway closure.

Once upper airway swelling begins, it often progresses so rapidly that passage of an ET tube (orally or nasally) through the edematous vocal cords may be extremely difficult, if not impossible, to perform. Prompt intubation, before the airway completely closes, will therefore be required in this child.

Because children have an inherently narrow airway, even a small amount of swelling can result in sufficient obstruction to cause inadequate ventilation, severe hypoxia, and respiratory failure.

Inhalation burn injuries to the airway are almost always confined to the upper airway structures, such as the oropharynx, nasopharynx, hypopharynx, and larynx. Because the upper airway is highly vascular and has a large surface area, hot inspired air or water vapor is quickly absorbed by the oropharynx and cooled to body temperature. Although this causes an immediate edematous response of the upper airway, the lower airway, including the lungs, remains relatively protected. Thermal injury to the lower airway is highly uncommon, occurring in only a fraction of patients who present with moderate to severe burns.

When burns occur to the neck and face, extravasation of plasma into the burned area can result in progressive edema and airway compromise as well. However, this usually does not occur until several hours after the burn; it is not often encountered in the prehospital setting.

Inhalation injury is present in 60% to 70% of all burn patients who die, making it the most common cause of burn-related deaths. In fact, the vast majority of burn-related deaths are caused by inhalation injury rather than the burn itself.

When a person is trapped in a smoke-filled environment, they inhale not only superheated air and steam, but other toxic substances as well, such as carbon monoxide (CO) and cyanide. The risk of inhalation injury is significantly higher if the patient lost consciousness while trapped. Unconscious patients have no control over their airway, nor can they control what they inhale (or don't inhale).

During the acute phase of burn patient management, upper airway swelling is the most immediate threat to the patient's life and often necessitates early intubation. Once this child's airway is secured with an ET tube, aggressive oxygenation and ventilation must be provided, based on the assumption that he has also experienced significant CO and cyanide exposure.

When assessing a burn patient, especially one who was entrapped and unconscious in a burning environment, the paramedic must closely monitor the patient for signs of upper airway inhalation injury (**Table 8-6**) and be prepared to perform intubation at once.

Table 8-6 Clinical Signs of Upper Airway Inhalation Injury

Carbonaceous (sooty) sputum in the mouth or nose
Singed nasal or facial hair
Hoarseness
Brassy-sounding cough
Visible facial burns
Stridor
Respiratory distress
Signs of hypoxemia

After preoxygenating the child with a bag-valve-mask device, follow these general guidelines when intubating a child with an inhalation burn injury to minimize the risk of airway damage and further supraglottic swelling:

- Use an ET tube that is 0.5 to 1 mm smaller than you would normally use.
- Avoid prolonged (> 20 seconds) or difficult intubation attempts.
- Consider nasotracheal intubation (if no contraindications exist).

If bag-valve-mask ventilations are not effective and intubation is not possible, a cricothyrotomy (needle or surgical) should be performed.

If the child with impending airway closure is conscious or semiconscious, intubation may need to be facilitated with pharmacological agents (eg, rapid sequence intubation [RSI]). Such pharmacological agents include benzodiazepines (eg, Versed, Valium) for sedation, and neuromuscular blockers (eg, succinylcholine, Norcuron) to induce paralysis. Follow locally established protocols or contact medical control as needed regarding RSI in children.

4. Why are burns more life-threatening in children than in adults?

Burns are a leading cause of death in children under 14 years of age. The child's survival depends on several factors, including the depth (degree) and extent of the burns, the presence of inhalation injury, and the presence of concomitant injury (eg, spinal trauma, head injury).

There are numerous reasons why burn injuries in children are more life-threatening than in an adult. Children have thinner skin that is more easily damaged; therefore, the same mechanism that would otherwise result in superficial burns in an adult could result in partial- or full-thickness burns in a child. Additionally, loss of the protective barrier that the skin provides significantly increases a child's risk of infection. Smaller children, whose immune systems are relatively immature to begin with, are especially prone to infection.

Children have a relatively large body surface area in proportion to their body weight, and because their heat-producing compensatory mechanisms (eg, shivering) are not well developed, they are at higher risk for hypothermia than adults are. Hypothermia will result in less effective resuscitative efforts (eg, fluid resuscitation, oxygenation) and will interfere with the process of hemostasis (the body's natural blood-clotting ability) if the patient is experiencing internal bleeding.

Because children have smaller fluid reserves than adults, they are more prone to dehydration and hypovolemic shock than adults. Even superficial (first degree) burns that cover a significant portion of a child's body can result in significant dehydration and shock.

As previously discussed, children are more prone to rapid upper airway swelling and closure because of their inherently narrow airways. Airway swelling may begin as soon as 30 minutes following an inhalation injury.

When assessing a child with a burn injury, the paramedic must keep these anatomic and physiologic differences in mind, especially if the child has experienced critical burns. In general, critically injured patients (including burn patients) should be transported to the closest trauma center for immediate stabilization. However, in certain cases, medical control may order you to transport the child to a specialized burn center.

The American Burn Association (ABA) categorizes burns as being mild, moderate, and severe, based on the depth (degree) of the burn, extent of the body surface area (BSA) burned, and age of the patient. **Table 8-7** summarizes the severity of burns in the pediatric patient and is based on the ABA burn severity categorization.

Table 8-7 Categorization of Pediatric Burn Severity

Minor burns
- Superficial and partial-thickness burns ≤ 10% BSA
- Full-thickness burns ≤ 2% BSA
- No burns to the hands, feet, face, or genitalia
- No concomitant trauma or significant underlying medical problems

Moderate burns
- Mixed partial- and full-thickness burns of 10% to 20% BSA
- Full-thickness burns ≤ 10% BSA
- No burns to the hands, feet, face, or genitalia
- No concomitant trauma or significant underlying medical problems

Severe burns
- All burns affecting ≥ 20% BSA
- Full-thickness burns ≥ 10% BSA
- All burns involving the hands, feet, face, and genitalia
- Circumferential burns of the chest or an extremity
- Electrical, chemical, and inhalation burns
- Concomitant trauma (eg, head injury, fractures)
- Preexisting serious underlying medical illness (eg, diabetes, asthma, heart disease)
- Burns that occur in high-risk patients (eg, infants, elderly)

5. What is the appropriate IV fluid therapy for this child?

Early fluid loss and hypovolemic shock are more common in children than in adults following a burn injury. This child is clearly experiencing hypovolemic shock, as evidenced by the following clinical signs:

- Tachycardia
- Weak peripheral pulses
- Delayed capillary refill
- Cool and pale skin

In order to maintain adequate perfusion, administer 20-mL/kg boluses of an isotonic crystalloid solution, such as normal saline or lactated Ringer's solution. Additional fluid boluses should be repeated if there is no response to the initial bolus.

Of particular concern with the burn patient is the presence of burn shock. Burn shock is a specific type of hypovolemic shock that typically occurs within the first 8 to 12 hours following the burn. During burn shock, fluid progressively shifts from the vascular compartment to the burned areas, resulting in inadequate systemic perfusion.

If your transport time will be in excess of 30 minutes, medical control may order continuous fluid replacement to prevent or minimize the effects of burn shock. The Parkland formula is the most commonly used method for calculating the appropriate fluid replacement for a burn patient. Because the greatest amount of plasma loss occurs in the first 24 hours following a severe burn (often sooner in children), aggressive fluid replacement must also occur during this time frame.

The Parkland formula determines how much fluid the patient should receive during the first 24 hours following the burn, and is calculated as follows:

4 mL × body weight in kg × % BSA burned = 24-hour fluid replacement

To determine how much fluid this child should receive, you must first estimate his weight in kilograms (kg). If the child's exact weight is unknown, use the following formula:

$$\text{Age (in years)} \times 2 + 8 = \text{weight in kg}$$

On the basis of the above formula, an average 9-year-old child weighs approximately 26 kilograms (9 [age in years] × 2 = 18 + 8 = 26 kg).

Next, using his BSA burns (39%), calculate how much IV fluid he should receive during the first 24 hours following the burn:

$$4 \text{ mL} \times 26 \text{ (kg)} \times 39 \text{ (\% BSA burned)} = 4,056 \text{ mL (over 24 hours)}$$

The Parkland formula further states that half of the 24-hour fluid volume should be given during the first 8 hours following the burn. Therefore, the calculation continues as follows:

- 4,056 mL ÷ 2 = 2,028 mL per 8 hours
- 2,028 mL ÷ 8 = 254 mL per hour

Using a macrodrip IV tubing (10 gtts/mL), this child's maintenance IV should therefore be set to run at *42 drops per minute (gtts/min)*:

$$254 \text{ mL} \times 10 \text{ (gtts/mL)} \div 60 \text{ (total hours [in minutes])} = 42 \text{ drops per minute}$$

It should be emphasized that the Parkland formula (or similar formulas) would not be appropriate for a child in hypovolemic shock and impending cardiovascular collapse. Instead, 20 mL/kg crystalloid fluid boluses, repeated as needed, would be indicated.

Summary

Approximately 1.2 million Americans experience burns each year. Of the nearly 51,000 patients admitted to hospitals each year for care of their burns, approximately 5,500 of them will die. Burns are the second leading cause of unintentional death in children between 1 and 4 years of age, and the third leading cause of injury and death in children between 1 and 18 years of age.

Burns, which occur when the body absorbs more heat that it can effectively dissipate, are classified as being superficial (first degree), partial-thickness (second degree), and full-thickness (third degree). Children, because of their thin skin, often experience more significant burns by the same mechanism that would otherwise cause less severe burns in the adult.

Early death from burns is usually the result of inhalation injury (eg, CO or cyanide toxicity, airway swelling), rather than the burn itself. Inhalation injury is most likely to occur when a patient is trapped in a burning environment, especially if there is an associated loss of consciousness. Late death is typically caused by massive infection and/or multiple organ failure.

Initial management for the burn patient begins by ensuring your own safety. Move the patient to a safe place and stop the burning process, if it is still occurring. Quickly assess the patient's airway, breathing, and circulatory status and intervene as needed. If the mechanism of injury is unclear, full spinal motion restriction precautions should be taken.

Because of rapid upper airway swelling, early intubation may be required—especially in children, whose airway is inherently small and prone to closure with even slight swelling. Pharmacological agents (eg, RSI) may be needed to facilitate intubation in a conscious or semiconscious child, who would otherwise not tolerate laryngoscopy and ET tube insertion.

Because of their relatively smaller fluid reserves, children are more prone to hypovolemic shock than the adult, and will require 20 mL/kg boluses of an isotonic crystalloid in order to maintain adequate perfusion and prevent cardiovascular collapse. Continual IV fluid replacement (eg, Parkland formula) may be required if transport times are lengthy, or if ordered by medical control.

The child's proportionately large BSA-to-weight ratio significantly increases the risk of hypothermia following a significant burn. Therefore, thermal management is a critical aspect of pediatric burn care, as it is with any patient.

Because of hypoxia and the inhalation of toxic gases, continuous monitoring of the child's cardiac rhythm is essential. You must be prepared to treat arrhythmias should they occur. Follow standard Pediatric Advanced Life Support (PALS) treatment algorithms when treating arrhythmias and cardiac arrest. The patient's oxygen saturation should also be continuously monitored. However, because the pulse oximeter may not be able to distinguish oxyhemoglobin (association of hemoglobin molecules and red blood cells) from carboxyhemoglobin (association of CO molecules and red blood cells), it can produce a falsely high reading in cases of carbon monoxide toxicity.

Specific burn management includes covering all burns (regardless of depth) with dry, sterile dressings, and avoiding the application of burn creams or ointments. Consider narcotic analgesic medications (eg, morphine, fentanyl citrate, Nubain) for pain relief in hemodynamically stable patients. Naloxone (Narcan) should be available to counteract the CNS depressant effects of narcotics (eg, respiratory depression, hypotension, bradycardia), should they occur.

In general, all critically injured patients should be rapidly transported to the closest trauma center, including burn patients. However, medical control may order you to transport the critically burned child directly to a burn center. Follow locally established protocols or contact medical control as needed regarding the treatment and transport of the burned child.

9

6-Month-Old Male in Respiratory Distress

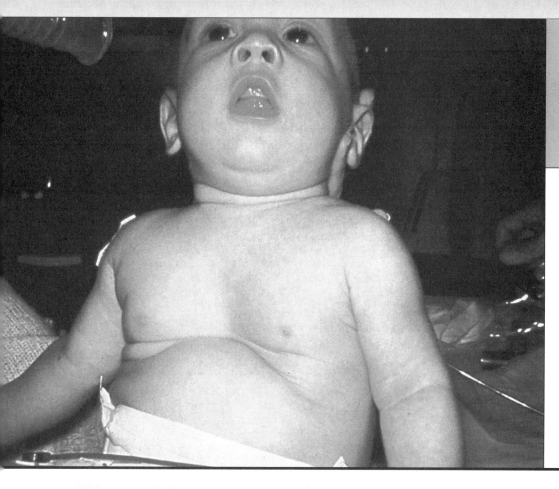

You are dispatched to 6401 West Brownsmith Street for a 6-month-old male with respiratory distress. The time of the call is 8:45 PM, and the temperature outside is 30°F. You proceed to the scene, with a response time of approximately 8 minutes.

You arrive at the scene at 8:53 PM and are met at the door of the residence by the infant's mother, who is holding her child. You note that the ill-appearing infant is in obvious respiratory distress, is coughing, and has a runny nose. After sitting the mother on the couch, you perform an initial assessment of the infant (**Table 9-1**).

Table 9-1 Initial Assessment

Level of Consciousness	Conscious, decreased interactiveness
Chief Complaint	Respiratory distress
Airway and Breathing	Airway is patent; respirations, rapid and labored; nasal flaring is present.
Circulation	Brachial pulse, rapid and strong; skin, warm and dry; capillary refill time, 2 seconds

Your partner hands the mother an oxygen mask to hold near the infant's face as you perform a focused history and physical examination (**Table 9-2**). The infant's mother states that she called 9-1-1 when her son suddenly stopped crying and turned blue. After she picked the infant up, however, the episode resolved. She also tells you that the infant was premature; he was born at 30 weeks' gestation.

Table 9-2 Focused History and Physical Examination

Onset	"He has had a cough and runny nose for the last 2 days; but then he started having trouble breathing, which has gradually worsened."
Severity	Marked intercostal retractions and nasal flaring are noted during inspiration.
Time of Onset	"He began having trouble breathing this morning, about 8 hours ago."
Associated Symptoms	Low-grade fever (101.5°F), poor feeding
Interventions Prior to EMS Arrival	"I suctioned his nose three times to try to keep it clear."

1. What is the likely cause of this infant's respiratory distress?

_____

_____

_____

You auscultate the infant's lungs and hear expiratory wheezing and coarse rhonchi bilaterally. With blow-by oxygen, the infant's oxygen saturation is 92%. As you open the medication box in preparation for further treatment, your partner attaches the cardiac monitor and assesses the infant's cardiac rhythm (**Figure 9-1**).

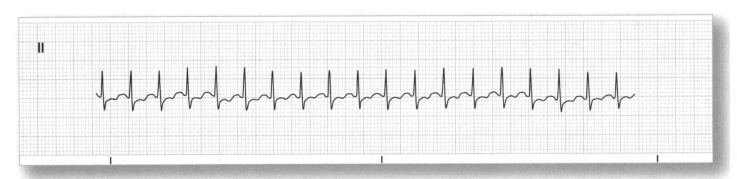

■ **Figure 9-1** The infant's cardiac rhythm.

2. What specific treatment is indicated for this infant's condition?

_____

_____

_____

_____

The infant's condition remains unchanged following your treatment. His level of alertness has decreased and his respirations have become slow and shallow. You look at the pulse oximeter and it reads 86%.

3. How will you manage this infant's deteriorating condition?

_____

_____

_____

_____

You quickly move the infant to the ambulance and continue further treatment. Despite your interventions, the infant's condition continues to deteriorate. His oxygen saturation continues to fall and the cardiac monitor now displays sinus bradycardia at 70 beats/min. Following your protocol, you prepare to perform rapid sequence intubation.

4. How is rapid sequence intubation performed in the infant?

_____

_____

_____

_____

Your attempts to obtain IV access in the infant's hands and feet are unsuccessful. After placing an intraosseous cannula in the infant's proximal tibia, you administer the necessary medications and successfully intubate the infant. You attach an automatic transport ventilator (ATV), set the tidal volume and ventilatory rate accordingly, and proceed to a hospital located 20 miles away. En route, you perform an ongoing assessment (**Table 9-3**) and then call your radio report to the receiving facility.

Table 9-3 Ongoing Assessment

Level of Consciousness	Sedated and paralyzed with neuromuscular blockade
Airway and Breathing	Intubated; ventilated at a rate of 20 breaths/min
Oxygen Saturation	96% (ventilated with 100% oxygen)
Heart Rate	120 beats/min, strong and regular
Capillary Refill Time	2 seconds
Digital Capnometry	36 mm Hg

The infant's condition has improved during transport. You arrive at the emergency department and give your verbal report to the attending physician. After further assessment and treatment in the emergency department, the infant is admitted to the pediatric ICU, where a pediatrician cares for him. Following resolution of his illness, the infant recovered and was later discharged home.

1. What is the likely cause of this infant's respiratory distress?

In addition to the obvious respiratory distress, the following environmental and clinical findings suggest that this infant is experiencing *bronchiolitis*:

- Cold ambient temperature
- Age less than 2 years
- Recent cough and congestion
- Runny nose (rhinorrhea)
- Low-grade fever
- Preterm gestation

Bronchiolitis is a viral infection of the bronchioles in the lower airway. It most commonly affects children less than 2 years of age and has a higher rate of occurrence during the winter months.

Any number of viruses can cause bronchiolitis, including influenza type A, parainfluenza, metapneumovirus, and adenovirus. However, many cases of bronchiolitis are caused by the respiratory syncytial virus (RSV). Unless the infant is very young with an immature immune system, most children develop life-long immunity to RSV following infection.

Infants less than 2 months of age are at greatest risk for developing respiratory failure secondary to bronchiolitis, especially if there is an associated history of prematurity, underlying pulmonary disease, or immune deficiency.

Bronchiolitis results in destruction of the lining of the bronchioles, profuse secretions, and bronchoconstriction. Infants are especially predisposed to bronchiolitis and respiratory failure because of their narrow airway size, high resistance to airflow, and decreased ability to clear their airway with an effective cough.

Bronchiolitis has a clinical presentation that can be similar to that of asthma. However, unlike bronchiolitis, asthma does not have a seasonal preponderance and is usually not accompanied by fever. **Table 9-4** illustrates the differential diagnosis of bronchiolitis and asthma. A major distinguishing factor in differentiating bronchiolitis from asthma is the child's age. Asthma rarely occurs before 1 year of age, whereas bronchiolitis is highly common in this age group.

Table 9-4 Differential Diagnosis of Bronchiolitis and Asthma

Clinical Findings	Bronchiolitis	Asthma
Age	< 2 years of age	> 1 year of age
Season	Winter	Any time
History of asthma	None	Present
Fever	Present	Usually none
Etiology	Virus	Often allergic
Resolution with beta-agonist	Variable	Yes
Breath Sounds	Diffuse, coarse rhonchi	Wheezing

Bronchiolitis is typically self-limiting and relatively benign; however, if left untreated, respiratory failure could develop, especially in high-risk infants. Assessment of the child with bronchiolitis commonly reveals varying degrees of increased work of breathing, tachypnea, wheezing, and tachycardia.

When assessing the child with suspected bronchiolitis, the paramedic must closely observe for clinical predictors of respiratory failure (**Table 9-5**) and be prepared to initiate aggressive management. Untreated or inappropriately treated respiratory failure may progress to cardiopulmonary arrest.

Table 9-5 Clinical Predictors of Respiratory Failure in Suspected Bronchiolitis

Early signs (compensating)
- Tachypnea (respirations > 60 breaths/min)
- Increased work of breathing
  - Intercostal or sternal retractions
  - Tracheal tugging
  - Nasal flaring
- Tachycardia (heart rate > 200 beats/min)
- Oxygen saturation of 90% to 94%
  - Indicates mild to moderate hypoxemia

Late signs (decompensating/impending respiratory failure)
- Bradypnea (respirations < 20 breaths/min)
- Decreased work of breathing
  - Decreased retractions
  - Shallow breathing (reduced tidal volume)
  - Signs of physical exhaustion
- Bradycardia (heart rate < 80 beats/min)
- Oxygen saturation less than 90% despite supplemental oxygen
  - Indicates severe hypoxemia

2. What specific treatment is indicated for this infant's condition?

After suctioning the nose and mouth to facilitate airway patency and adequate ventilation, administer 100% humidified oxygen via pediatric nonrebreathing mask or with the blow-by technique. Humidified oxygen will help loosen thick lower airway secretions, making them easier for the child to expel. Intubation and ventilation equipment should be readily available if the child develops respiratory failure and apnea.

To relieve bronchoconstriction, two medications may be helpful: albuterol and racemic epinephrine. The dose of albuterol for children less than 15 kg (33 lb) is 2.5 to 5 mg (0.5–1 mL of a 0.5% solution). Dilute the albuterol in 3 mL of normal saline and administer it via small-volume nebulizer. This dose can be repeated every 20 minutes, up to 3 doses.

Infants are obviously not able to use a nebulizer as an older child would; therefore, hold the device near the infant's nose and mouth, allowing him or her to breathe the nebulized medication.

The dose of racemic epinephrine is 0.25 mg (0.25 mL) of the 2.25% solution for children < 10 kg and 0.5 mg (0.5 mL) of the 2.25% solution for children > 10 kg. Racemic epinephrine should also be given via nebulizer and should also be diluted in 3 mL of normal saline.

If the infant's respirations are ineffective (eg, reduced tidal volume), bronchodilator therapy can be administered in conjunction with bag-valve-mask ventilations, using a small-volume inline nebulizer.

The lower airway obstruction associated with bronchiolitis is caused by two factors: bronchoconstriction and copious, thick mucous secretions. Because the primary pathology of asthma is bronchoconstriction, nebulized beta₂ agonists usually produce marked improvement, if not complete resolution, of the child's symptoms. However, only partial improvement may be seen in children with bronchiolitis following the administration of beta₂ agonists because they are effective in relieving bronchoconstriction, but are ineffective in removing the secretions from the lower airway.

Additional treatment for bronchiolitis includes continuous monitoring of the child's cardiac rhythm and oxygen saturation. If little or no relief is seen following nebulized bronchodilators, and the child's condition begins to worsen, prepare to perform assisted ventilations and, if necessary, endotracheal intubation.

3. How will you manage this infant's deteriorating condition?

■ Positive-pressure ventilatory assistance

Because of progressive hypoxia and prolonged increased work of breathing, this infant has become physically exhausted and is no longer able to effectively compensate for his condition. Therefore, you must initiate assisted ventilations with a bag-valve-mask device and 100% oxygen in order to restore adequate minute volume and prevent respiratory arrest.

To maximize the effectiveness of ventilations, ensure that the infant's head is correctly positioned, use an appropriate-sized mask, and suction oral and nasal secretions as needed.

Because of the thick lower airway secretions associated with bronchiolitis, you may meet resistance when attempting ventilations. If the pediatric bag-valve-mask device you are using is equipped with a pop-off release valve, it should be occluded in order to allow you to achieve adequate tidal volume. However, you should exercise caution when ventilating the child; overzealous ventilation may cause barotrauma and a resultant pneumothorax.

4. How is rapid sequence intubation performed in the infant?

Rapid sequence intubation (RSI) involves the administration of both a potent sedative-hypnotic agent and a neuromuscular blocking agent (paralytic) to facilitate intubation, while minimizing the risks of aspiration and potential harm to the patient. Other medications may be used in conjunction with RSI as dictated by the patient's age and clinical condition. RSI should be considered when a patient, whose level of consciousness would otherwise contraindicate intubation (eg, combative, semiconscious), is clinically unstable and requires definitive airway management.

RSI is used widely in the emergency department when critically ill or injured patients require intubation; it is also becoming increasingly popular in the prehospital setting. RSI is an effective means of definitively securing and maintaining a patent airway, especially when the patient requires prolonged ventilatory support or transport time to the hospital is prolonged. It should be noted, however, that if the patient's airway can be *effectively* managed by other, less invasive means, RSI would not be appropriate.

Although the medications used may vary slightly in each EMS system, the following sequence is a generally recommended approach to performing RSI on an infant:

1. Preoxygenate the infant.
2. Obtain IV access (if not already done).
   • Place an intraosseous (IO) cannula if IV access is unsuccessful after three attempts *or* 90 seconds.
3. Prepare the necessary equipment and medications.
4. Attach a cardiac monitor and pulse oximeter.

5. Premedicate
- Atropine 0.02 mg/kg (minimum dose of 0.1 mg)
  - Indicated in children less than 5 years of age
  - Indicated in *all* children when succinylcholine (Anectine) is used

Premedication with atropine blocks the reflex bradycardia associated with the use of succinylcholine and laryngoscopy. This reflex is more pronounced in children under 5 years of age. To maximize the effectiveness of atropine, it should be administered at least 2 minutes prior to intubation.

6. Sedate (use **one** of the following)
- Midazolam (Versed) 0.1 to 0.2 mg/kg
  - Maximum of 4 mg
- Diazepam (Valium) 0.1 to 0.2 mg/kg
  - Maximum of 4 mg
- Etomidate (Amidate) 0.2 to 0.4 mg/kg

If a benzodiazepine such as midazolam or diazepam is used, an opiate such as fentanyl (2 µg/kg IV) or morphine (0.1 mg/kg IV) should be used in conjunction with it for intubation. The above sedative-hypnotic medications represent those commonly used in the prehospital setting. Other medications may be used as authorized by local protocol or medical control.

7. Neuromuscular blocker (use **one** of the following)
- Succinylcholine 2 mg/kg
  - 15 to 30 second onset of action; 3- to 5-minute duration of action
  - Do not use in patients with a history of muscular dystrophy, cerebral palsy, or conditions that may cause high potassium levels (eg, renal failure).
- Rocuronium bromide (Zemuron) 0.6 to 1.2 mg/kg
  - 15 to 30 second onset of action; 30- to 60-minute duration of action
  - Minimal cardiovascular side effects

Other neuromuscular blocking medications may be used for RSI in children; refer to your local protocol as needed.

8. Apply cricoid pressure.

9. Perform endotracheal intubation.
- Confirm correct ET tube placement by auscultation and capnography.
- Properly secure the ET tube.
- Ventilate the infant at the appropriate rate.

10. Observe and monitor.
- Administer additional sedation and paralytics as needed.

RSI should *only* be attempted by properly trained paramedics, who are authorized to perform the procedure by direct medical control or local protocol. Familiarity with the medications used during RSI and proficiency at intubation are crucial.

Once the patient has been medicated (ie, they are paralyzed), the paramedic must be able to secure the patient's airway. If intubation is unsuccessful, the paramedic must have an alternate means of securing a patent airway.

Summary
Bronchiolitis, a viral infection of the lower airway, is a common respiratory illness in children under 2 years of age. It is characterized by bronchospasm, thick lower airway secretions, and low-grade fever. Bronchiolitis commonly occurs during the winter months.

Bronchiolitis is usually self-limited and relatively benign; however, if left untreated, varying degrees of increased work of breathing and hypoxemia can result. In severe cases, the child with bronchiolitis can develop respiratory failure.

Initial management for the child with bronchiolitis includes establishing a patent airway and ensuring adequate oxygenation and ventilation. Beta$_2$ agonists such as albuterol or racemic epinephrine may provide improvement in the child's respiratory distress by increasing the patency of the bronchioles and improving ventilation. Humidified oxygen, either by nonrebreathing mask or the blow-by method, may help loosen secretions in the lower airway, making them easier for the child to expel.

In some cases, the infant or child with bronchiolitis may develop respiratory failure and require assisted ventilations with a bag-valve-mask device and 100% oxygen. Infants less than 2 months of age have the greatest risk for developing respiratory failure secondary to bronchiolitis, especially if there is an associated history of prematurity, underlying pulmonary disease, or immune deficiency.

If the child's condition continues to deteriorate despite properly performed bag-valve-mask ventilations and 100% oxygen, endotracheal intubation should be considered. In the conscious or semiconscious child, sedation and neuromuscular blocking medications are usually needed in order to facilitate placement of the ET tube. In children less than 5 years of age, premedication with atropine may decrease the incidence of bradycardia associated with laryngoscopy and succinylcholine.

Ensuring adequate oxygenation and ventilation are crucial in the management of an infant or child with respiratory failure. Failure of the respiratory system is the most common cause of cardiopulmonary arrest in children.

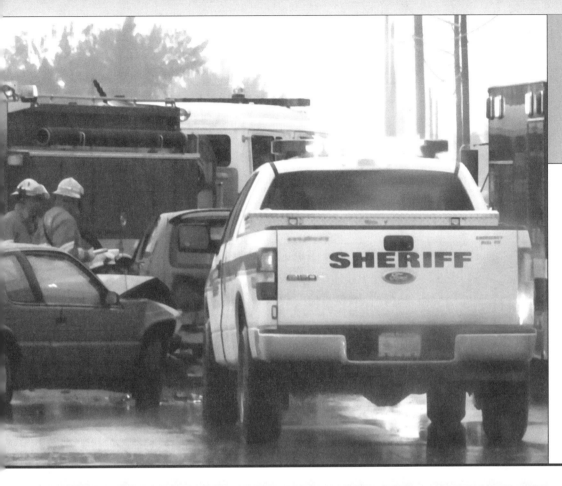

5-Year-Old Male Involved in a Motor Vehicle Crash

At 4:35 PM, you receive a call for a head-on collision involving two passenger cars. Your unit and a fire department rescue unit are dispatched simultaneously, with a response time to the scene of approximately 5 minutes.

Your unit and the rescue unit arrive at the scene simultaneously. The driver of the first vehicle appears uninjured and refuses EMS care. The driver of the second vehicle, a young female, has minor injuries and also refuses EMS care. She is holding her child, a 5-year-old male, screaming for you to help him. The child was unrestrained in the back seat and apparently thrust into the back of the passenger seat upon impact. He is conscious and alert, but in obvious respiratory distress. The child is placed onto a long spine board, and, as your partner maintains stabilization of his head, you perform an initial assessment (**Table 10-1**).

Table 10-1 Initial Assessment

Mechanism of Injury	Head-on motor vehicle crash at 40 MPH, unrestrained
Level of Consciousness	Conscious and crying; restless
Chief Complaint	Respiratory distress
Airway and Breathing	Airway is patent; respirations, increased and labored
Circulation	Radial pulses, rapid and regular; skin, cool and moist; capillary refill time, 2 seconds; no gross bleeding

1. On the basis of the mechanism of injury and initial assessment findings, what is your impression of this child?

_____

_____

_____

You place the child on 100% oxygen with a nonrebreathing mask. As a rescue team member retrieves a cervical collar, head blocks, and straps from the ambulance, you perform a rapid trauma assessment on the child (**Table 10-2**).

Table 10-2 Rapid Trauma Assessment

Head	No obvious trauma; no gross bleeding
Neck	Trachea is midline; jugular veins appear normal
Chest	Abrasion to the right side of the chest; chest wall is stable with no deformities or crepitus; breath sounds diminished on the right
Abdomen/Pelvis	Abdomen is soft and non-tender; pelvis, stable
Lower Extremities	No obvious trauma; pedal pulses, bilaterally present; sensory and motor functions, grossly intact
Upper Extremities	No obvious trauma; radial pulses, bilaterally present; sensory and motor functions, grossly intact
Posterior	No obvious trauma

2. What type of injury should you suspect this child to be experiencing?

_____

_____

_____

_____

Full spinal motion restriction precautions are applied and the child is quickly loaded into the ambulance. You obtain baseline vital signs and a SAMPLE history (**Table 10-3**) as your partner prepares the supplies to start an IV. The child remains conscious; however, he is becoming increasingly restless and dyspneic. The child's mother provides information regarding her son's medical history.

Table 10-3 Baseline Vital Signs and SAMPLE History

Blood Pressure	92/58 mm Hg
Pulse	130 beats/min, strong and regular
Capillary Refill Time	3 seconds
Respirations	40 breaths/min and labored
Oxygen Saturation	93% (on 100% oxygen)
Signs and Symptoms	Chest wall abrasions, unilaterally diminished breath sounds, tachypnea, dyspnea, tachycardia
Allergies	None
Medications	None
Pertinent Past History	None
Last Oral Intake	"We had lunch about 3 hours ago."
Events Leading to Injury	"I was talking on my cellular phone, when I hit the car coming toward me."

Transport to a trauma center, which is located 15 miles away, is begun. The child's mother accompanies her son in the ambulance. En route, you establish an IV of normal saline with a 20-gauge catheter and attach the cardiac monitor, which reveals a sinus tachycardia at 160 beats/min. You reassess the child and note that his level of consciousness has decreased. His respirations have become markedly labored and chest wall movement appears asymmetrical. Despite 100% oxygen, his oxygen saturation reads 86%.

3. Why is this child's condition deteriorating? How will you intervene?

_____

_____

_____

_____

Following the appropriate intervention, you note improvement in the child's condition. His respiratory effort has improved and his oxygen saturation now reads 97%. Further reassessment reveals that his skin color and condition have improved and his heart rate has decreased to 120 beats/min.

4. Does this child require IV crystalloid fluid boluses?

_____

_____

_____

_____

As you continue to reassess the child, you note that breath sounds on the right side of his chest, although still somewhat diminished, are audible and chest wall movement is symmetrical. With an estimated time of arrival at the trauma center of 5 minutes, you perform an ongoing assessment (**Table 10-4**) and then call your radio report to the receiving facility.

Table 10-4 Ongoing Assessment

Level of Consciousness	Conscious and alert, crying, less restless
Airway and Breathing	Airway remains patent; respirations, 24 breaths/min with adequate depth
Oxygen Saturation	98% (on 100% oxygen)
Blood Pressure	90/56 mm Hg
Pulse	114 beats/min, strong and regular
Capillary Refill Time	1 to 2 seconds
ECG	Normal sinus rhythm

The child's condition continues to improve during the remainder of the transport. You arrive at the trauma center and give your verbal report to the attending physician. After further assessment and treatment in the emergency department, the child is admitted to the pediatric ICU where he later recovered and was discharged home.

1. On the basis of the mechanism of injury and initial assessment findings, what is your impression of this child?

A crucial part of the scene size-up involves closely examining the mechanism of injury (MOI). The MOI will help you predict possible injuries that the patient may have sustained at the time of impact. There are two significant findings with this particular MOI that should increase your index of suspicion for possible serious injury:

- **Rapid deceleration from 40 MPH**

- **Lack of restraint use**

Although serious injuries may occur at lower speeds, speeds greater than 35 MPH at the time of impact are more likely to result in life-threatening injuries. Head-on collisions occur when the forward momentum of a car stops abruptly (rapid deceleration), such as when it strikes another car traveling in the opposite direction or strikes a fixed object such as a tree or bridge pillar. It is important to note that with this type of MOI, three separate collisions occur:

- **Collision of the car against another moving car or fixed object**

Mass (weight) and velocity (speed) are converted into kinetic energy (force). In the case of a head-on motor vehicle crash, the kinetic energy of the moving car is converted into the work of stopping the car, usually by crushing the car's exterior. Although damage to the exterior of the vehicle is often the most dramatic part of the collision, it does not directly affect patient care. It does, however, provide information about the severity of the collision and therefore has an indirect effect on patient care. The greater the damage to the vehicle, the greater the energy involved, and therefore the greater potential for serious injury to the passengers.

- **Collision of the passenger against the interior of the vehicle**

Just as the kinetic energy produced by the vehicle's mass and velocity is converted into the work of stopping the vehicle, the kinetic energy produced by the passenger's mass and velocity is converted into the work of stopping his or her body. And just like the obvious damage to the exterior of the vehicle, the injuries that result from this second collision may be dramatic and are often evident during your initial assessment of the patient. Your patient, who was unrestrained in the back seat at the time of impact, could have experienced a variety of injuries when he struck the back of the passenger's seat. You should be suspicious for head, chest, spine, and abdominal trauma.

- **Collision of the passenger's internal organs against the solid structures of the body**

Injuries that occur during the third collision may not be as obvious as external injuries caused by the second collision; however, they may be the most life-threatening. For example, as the passenger's head impacts a fixed object, the brain continues to move forward until it strikes the inside of the skull. This may result in compression injuries to the frontal aspect of the brain and stretching (or tearing) injuries to the occipital aspect of the brain. Although spinal injuries are less common in children than in adults, the cervical spine is less stable, and could have been injured as the child was thrust against the seat.

When the chest strikes a fixed object, the heart impacts the sternum and may cause myocardial contusion or rupture, resulting in life-threatening internal hemorrhage. Additionally, shearing injuries may occur to the aorta or vena cava, also resulting in life-threatening internal hemorrhage.

Your initial assessment findings reveal tachycardia, diaphoresis, and restlessness, indicating early shock. Additionally, the presence of respiratory distress suggests chest trauma. Although the absence of gross bleeding suggests blunt chest trauma, a rapid trauma assessment must be performed in order to detect other, potentially life-threatening injuries.

A child's ribs are softer and more flexible than an adult's; therefore, rib fractures are less likely to occur. However, the pliable ribcage may compress the lungs and heart, resulting in serious internal injuries (ie, pneumothorax or myocardial and pulmonary contusions) but little or no obvious evidence of external injury (**Figure 10-1**).

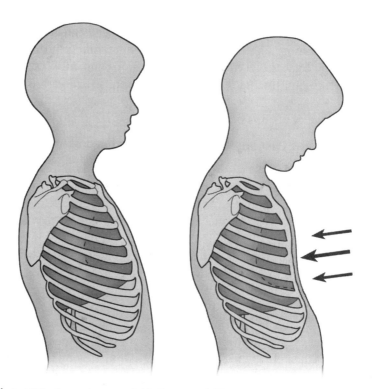

■ **Figure 10-1** A child's ribcage is more pliable than an adult's. As a result, compression injuries to the chest may occur without obvious external signs of injury.

2. What type of injury should you suspect this child to be experiencing?

On the basis of the following clinical findings, you should suspect that this child is experiencing a closed (simple) pneumothorax:

■ Respiratory distress

■ Unilaterally diminished breath sounds

■ External signs of blunt chest injury (eg, abrasions)

A pneumothorax occurs when air accumulates in between the visceral and parietal pleura, converting the potential pleural space to an actual one and progressively collapsing the lung. Pneumothorax can occur as the result of blunt or penetrating trauma to the chest (**Figure 10-2**).

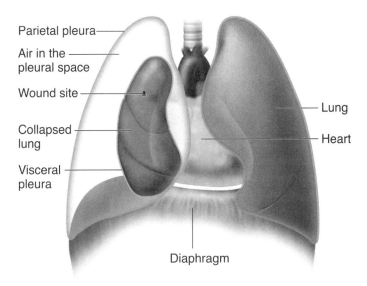

Parietal pleura

Air in the
pleural space

Wound site

Lung

Collapsed
lung

Heart

Visceral
pleura

Diaphragm

■ **Figure 10-2** Pneumothorax occurs when air leaks into the pleural space between the pleural surfaces from an opening in the chest wall (penetrating injury) or the surface of the lung (blunt injury). The lung collapses as air fills the pleural space.

With blunt chest trauma, rapid compression of the inflated lung may perforate the lung parenchyma and allow air to leak into the pleural space. This mechanism is referred to as the "paper bag" effect, because it is similar to an inflated paper bag that explodes when sudden force is exerted on it.

Another common cause of pneumothorax associated with blunt trauma is a fractured rib perforating the lung. Although this is a less likely cause of pneumothorax in a 5-year-old child, it is more common in adolescents and adults, whose ribs are less pliable and more prone to fracture.

Air in the pleural space will prevent the affected lung from expanding, thus reducing pulmonary capacity and effective gas exchange. The clinical presentation of a patient with a pneumothorax depends on the size of the pulmonary defect and the rate at which air is accumulating in the pleural space.

Classically, the patient with a pneumothorax presents with diminished breath sounds on the same side as the injury, restlessness, and varying degrees of tachypnea and respiratory distress. As the pneumothorax progresses, respirations become more labored, signs of shock develop (eg, tachycardia, delayed capillary refill, tachypnea), and oxygen saturation begins to fall. Percussion over the affected hemithorax may reveal hyperresonance; however, this is very difficult to assess in the field, particularly in infants and small children.

Because of damage to the lung and associated internal hemorrhage, some pneumothoraces are complicated by the presence of blood in the pleural space—a condition called hemopneumothorax. The signs and symptoms of hemopneumothorax are similar to those of a pneumothorax. In cases of massive hemopneumothorax, the patient presents with severe shock from internal hemorrhage, collapsed jugular veins, and profound respiratory distress.

3. Why is this child's condition deteriorating? How will you intervene?

This child's deteriorating condition suggests the progression of his simple pneumothorax to a tension pneumothorax. A tension pneumothorax occurs when pressure builds within the pleural space as the portion of the lung that is damaged acts as a one-way valve. This one-way-valve effect allows air to enter the pleural space but does not allow it to escape.

Increasing pressure within the pleural space further collapses the lung on the affected side and forces the mediastinum toward the unaffected side (**Figure 10-3**).

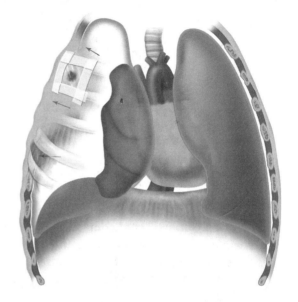

■ **Figure 10-3** A tension pneumothorax develops when air enters the pleural space but is not able to escape. This causes total collapse of the lung on the affected side and forces the mediastinum toward the unaffected side

As pressure shifts across the mediastinum, the heart, aorta, and vena cava are compressed, resulting in decreased preload and stroke volume and increased venous pressure.

The patient with a tension pneumothorax develops severe respiratory distress because the affected lung has completely collapsed, and, due to the mediastinal shift, is collapsing the unaffected lung as well. Breath sounds are usually absent on the affected side and may become diminished on the unaffected side. As the mediastinum shifts, tracheal deviation away from the affected side may be noted; however, this is a late sign. As tension exerts laterally, it is inhibited by the ribs, resulting in bulging of the intercostal muscles on the affected side.

Because of pressure on the myocardium and aorta, stroke volume and cardiac output are decreased, resulting in hypotension (obstructive shock). Tachycardia develops as a compensatory mechanism in response to the reduced cardiac output. Kinking of the vena cava causes decreased preload and increased venous pressure, which manifests clinically as distention of the external jugular veins. Narrowing of the pulse pressure may be seen and is caused when the myocardium is compressed, preventing effective cardiac contraction (systole) and inhibiting myocardial relaxation (diastole). This causes a decrease in systolic BP and an increase in diastolic BP. The signs and symptoms of a tension pneumothorax are summarized in **Table 10-5**.

Table 10-5 Signs and Symptoms of a Tension Pneumothorax

Severe respiratory distress
Absent breath sounds on the affected side
• Diminished breath sounds on the unaffected side
Asymmetrical chest movement
Bulging intercostals muscles on the affected side
Signs of shock:
• Restlessness
• Tachycardia
• Diaphoresis
• Hypotension (late sign)
Narrowing pulse pressure
Cyanosis
Low oxygen saturation
Jugular venous distention[1]
Tracheal deviation away from the affected side (late sign)[1]

[1] These signs may be undetectable in infants

Because infants and small children have small chests, breath sound differences from side to side may be more subtle than in older children and adults. Additionally, because of their short, fat necks, tracheal deviation and jugular venous distention may be undetectable. Tension pneumothorax should be suspected in the infant or child who has the following:

■ **Penetrating chest injury with respiratory distress, hypoxemia, and shock**

■ **Blunt chest trauma with respiratory distress, hypoxemia, and shock that worsens with assisted ventilation**
  • Oxygen-powered ventilation devices (eg, demand valve) are contraindicated in patients with chest trauma and in *all* children.

Although an inadequately breathing child requires assisted ventilation with 100% oxygen, if a tension pneumothorax is suspected, it is more crucial to perform immediate pleural decompression (needle thoracentesis). Continued assisted ventilation, especially in a small child, may cause faster progression of a simple pneumothorax to a tension pneumothorax.

Pleural decompression involves inserting a large-bore (14- or 16-gauge) IV catheter through the chest wall and into the pleural space. This will provide a port for air in the pleural space to escape, thus allowing the affected lung to re-expand and release tension from the unaffected lung, myocardium, and great vessels. Pleural decompression in the infant or child is performed in the second intercostal space at the mid-clavicular line (preferred) or in the fourth intercostal space at the anterior axillary line (**Figure 10-4**).

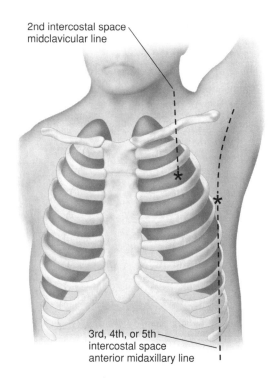

2nd intercostal space
midclavicular line

3rd, 4th, or 5th
intercostal space
anterior midaxillary line

■ **Figure 10-4** Pleural decompression can be performed in the second intercostal space at the midclavicular line (preferred) or in the fourth intercostal space at the anterior axillary line.

Attach a 14- or 16-gauge over-the-needle catheter to a 30-mL syringe. Before inserting the needle, count the ribs twice to ensure proper site location. The nipple line is usually at the fourth intercostal space. Follow these steps to perform pleural decompression in the infant or child:

1. Insert the needle through the skin at a 90° angle and advance until the tip hits a rib.

2. Advance the needle tip into the pleural space. A slight "pop" is usually felt when the needle pierces the outer pleural membrane (parietal pleura).

3. Pull back the plunger of the syringe to aspirate air.

4. Remove the syringe and stylet and leave the catheter in the pleural space, anchored in the chest wall.

5. Reassess the child, including rate and work of breathing, peripheral circulation, heart rate, and blood pressure.

Because intercostal blood vessels and nerves follow the inferior border of the rib, the needle should be inserted over the top of the rib margin to prevent causing injury to these structures (**Figure 10-5**).

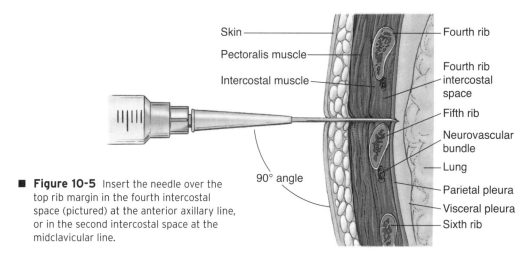

Skin

Pectoralis muscle

Intercostal muscle

90° angle

Fourth rib

Fourth rib intercostal space

Fifth rib

Neurovascular bundle

Lung

Parietal pleura

Visceral pleura

Sixth rib

■ **Figure 10-5** Insert the needle over the top rib margin in the fourth intercostal space (pictured) at the anterior axillary line, or in the second intercostal space at the midclavicular line.

Aspiration of air from the pleural space and improvement in the child's clinical condition confirm the presence of a tension pneumothorax. If no improvements in the child's work of breathing, heart rate, and skin perfusion are noted following pleural decompression, consider repeating the procedure on the contralateral side. Follow local protocol or contact medical control as needed regarding pleural decompression in the child.

Proper technique and identification of the correct anatomic landmarks are crucial when performing pleural decompression. Potential complications include open pneumothorax, hemothorax, diaphragm or bowel penetration (if performed at the fourth intercostal space), hemopericardium, and coronary vessel injury.

4. Does this child require IV crystalloid fluid boluses?

It is important to establish at least one IV line in any critically injured patient. Although internal bleeding cannot be totally ruled out in this child, improvement in his condition following pleural decompression suggests an obstructive etiology to his shock—not hypovolemia. Therefore, IV fluid boluses are not required at this point. Set the IV at a keep-vein-open rate and continue close monitoring until arrival at the hospital. If signs of hypovolemia develop (eg, pallor, poor peripheral perfusion, unlabored tachypnea), administer 20 mL/kg boluses of normal saline or lactated Ringer's solution to maintain perfusion.

Summary

This child's injury would most likely have been avoided had he been properly restrained in the backseat of the vehicle. Although he developed a tension pneumothorax, this injury can be treated in the prehospital setting. Many unrestrained children die each year as a result of motor vehicle crashes. Commonly, the child is propelled into the windshield, even from the backseat, and experiences massive head trauma.

Because the ribcage in a child is pliable, rib fracture and lung perforation is a relatively uncommon cause of pneumothorax. Most pneumothoraces in children are caused by either penetrating trauma or, when blunt trauma is involved, the "paper bag" effect previously discussed.

Signs and symptoms of a pneumothorax in children include varying degrees of tachypnea, increased work of breathing, and tachycardia. As tension builds within the pleural space, a contralateral shift in the mediastinum occurs, compressing the heart, aorta, and vena cava. As a tension pneumothorax develops, the child develops signs of shock and profound respiratory distress.

You should suspect a tension pneumothorax in a child with respiratory distress and hypoxemia following penetrating chest trauma. Following blunt chest trauma, worsened respiratory distress and hypoxemia, despite assisted ventilation, should also increase your suspicion of a tension pneumothorax.

Relative to adults, the signs and symptoms of a tension pneumothorax are less obvious in the infant or child. Because of their small chest wall, breath sound differences may be subtle from side to side. Additionally, jugular venous distention and tracheal deviation may be undetectable, especially in infants, whose necks are short and fat.

Emergency care for a child with a pneumothorax begins by ensuring a patent airway and adequate breathing. Administer 100% oxygen, apply full spinal motion restriction precautions as dictated by the mechanism of injury and promptly transport to a trauma center. Attempt to establish at least one IV, preferably en route to the hospital. If the child's condition deteriorates, pleural decompression will be necessary to release air from the pleural space and improve cardiopulmonary function.

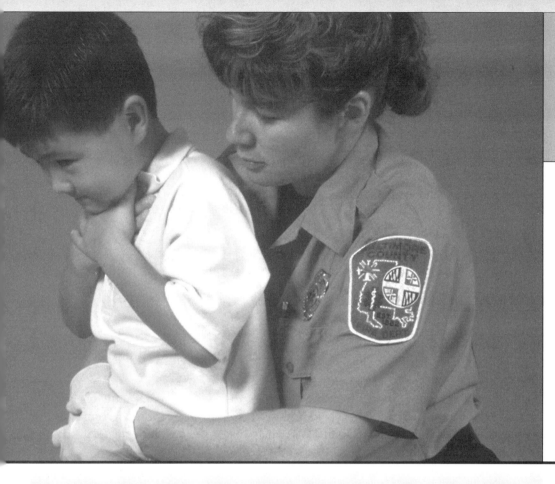

11

7-Year-Old Male with an Airway Obstruction

At 2:15 PM, you and your partner are sitting at the station watching TV when you hear a frantic knock at the door. As you approach the door, you hear a woman screaming "He's choking, please help me!"

Your partner runs to the ambulance to grab the jump kit as you perform an initial assessment on the child (Table 11-1). The child's mother tells you that he was eating a piece of hard candy when her car hit a large pothole in the road. When she looked at him to see if he was all right, he was grabbing his throat and was unable to talk.

Table 11-1 Initial Assessment

Level of Consciousness	Conscious; terrified look
Chief Complaint	Apparent airway obstruction
Airway and Breathing	Weakly audible cough, faint inspiratory stridor, minimal air movement at the nose and mouth
Circulation	Perioral cyanosis; radial pulse, rapid and strong; no gross bleeding

1. Does this child have good air exchange or poor air exchange? Why?

_____

_____

_____

_____

2. How will you manage this child's condition initially?

_____

_____

_____

Despite your initial attempts to treat the child's condition, he becomes unconscious, increasingly cyanotic, and apneic. As you place the child supine on the ground in preparation for further treatment, your partner prepares the bag-valve-mask device. The child's mother calls her husband and apprises him of the situation.

3. What is your next action in the management of this child?

_____

_____

_____

Several attempts to relieve the child's airway obstruction have failed. Your partner opens the advanced airway kit in preparation for further interventions. The child remains cyanotic and apneic. His pulse is still rapid; however, it is becoming weak.

4. What intervention is indicated now?

_____

_____

_____

You have successfully removed the piece of candy from the child's airway and are now able to ventilate him; however, he remains unconscious, cyanotic, and apneic. You palpate his carotid pulse and note that it is 65 beats/min. Additionally, his oxygen saturation reads 85%. Your partner quickly retrieves the stretcher from the ambulance in preparation for transport to a hospital located 30 miles away.

5. How will you continue to manage this child's condition?

_____

_____

_____

With your partner's assistance, the child's airway has been secured and ventilations are continued. He is quickly loaded into the ambulance, where you obtain baseline vital signs and a SAMPLE history (**Table 11-2**). The child's mother, who accompanies her son in the front seat of the ambulance, provides you with his medical information. En route to the hospital, you attach an automatic transport ventilator (ATV) and set the ventilatory rate and tidal volume accordingly.

Table 11-2 Baseline Vital Signs and SAMPLE History

Blood Pressure	90/50 mm Hg
Pulse	100 beats/min, strong and regular
Respirations	Intubated and ventilated at 20 breaths/min
Oxygen Saturation	97% (ventilated with 100% oxygen)
ECG	Normal sinus rhythm at 100 beats/min
Signs and Symptoms	Airway obstruction (relieved); unconscious, apneic
Allergies	None
Medications	Amoxicillin for a recent ear infection
Pertinent Past History	None
Last Oral Intake	"We ate lunch about 2 hours ago."
Events Leading to Present Illness	"He was eating a piece of hard candy and choked on it when I hit a pothole in the road."

During transport, you start an IV of normal saline with a 20-gauge catheter and continue to monitor the child's condition. You note that he is making occasional spontaneous efforts to breathe and is becoming restless, agitated, and somewhat resistant to the ET tube. His heart rate is 110 beats/min and his oxygen saturation is 99%. The digital capnometer reads 39 mm Hg.

6. Should you extubate this child? Why or why not?

Following the appropriate intervention, the child has calmed down and is no longer resisting the ET tube. With an estimated time of arrival at the hospital of 5 minutes, you perform an ongoing assessment (**Table 11-3**) and then ask your driver to call the radio report to the receiving facility.

Table 11-3 Ongoing Assessment

Level of Consciousness	Sedated; spontaneous movement of all extremities
Airway and Breathing	Occasional spontaneous respirations; intubated; ventilatory assistance is continued with a bag-valve-mask device and 100% oxygen.
Pulse	110 beats/min, strong and regular at the carotid artery
Blood Pressure	Unable to obtain; you are busy assisting the child's ventilations.
Oxygen Saturation	99% (assisted ventilation with 100% oxygen)
ECG	Normal sinus rhythm
Digital Capnometry	38 mm Hg

Upon arrival at the hospital, the child's condition has improved. He has regular, shallow respirations, which you are assisting with a bag-valve-mask device. You give your verbal report to the attending physician. An arterial blood gas reveals the following: pH, 7.40; PaO_2, 120 mm Hg; $PaCO_2$, 42 mm Hg; and SaO_2, 99%. A chest radiograph is obtained to rule out residual foreign bodies and the child is admitted to the pediatric ICU. Following a brief stay in the hospital, the child was discharged without neurologic deficit.

1. Does this child have good air exchange or poor air exchange? Why?

Although the child is conscious, the following clinical findings indicate that he has poor air exchange and thus, a severe airway obstruction:

- Weakly audible (ineffective) cough
- Faint inspiratory stridor
- Perioral cyanosis
- Minimal air movement at the nose and mouth

Foreign body upper airway obstructions are broadly classified as being mild or severe. Patients with a mild airway obstruction typically present with a sudden onset of respiratory distress, noisy respirations (ie, stridor, crowing), normal skin color, and a strong cough. They are able to exchange enough carbon dioxide and oxygen to maintain consciousness and their oxygen saturation is usually within normal limits (> 95%). *These patients should be left alone!* Encourage the patient to continue to cough, avoid agitation, provide supplemental oxygen as tolerated, and transport to the hospital. A strong, effective cough is the most effective means of clearing the airway. Attempts to relieve a mild airway obstruction may result in a severe airway obstruction.

Conscious patients with a severe airway obstruction cannot exchange enough carbon dioxide and oxygen to maintain consciousness or adequate oxygen saturation. Signs of a severe airway obstruction include an ineffective (weak) or absent cough, weak inspiratory stridor or crowing, cyanosis, decreasing level of consciousness, and decreasing oxygen saturation. Air movement at the nose and mouth is either minimal or absent. You must identify these patients quickly and take measures to relieve the obstruction before they lose consciousness. The characteristics of upper airway obstruction in the conscious patient are summarized in **Table 11-4**.

Table 11-4 Airway Obstruction in the Conscious Patient

Degree of Obstruction	Sound	Signs
Severe	Weak or absent	Severe anxiety, cyanosis, ineffective or absent cough, decreasing oxygen saturation, decreasing level of consciousness, minimal or no air movement
Mild	Noisy	Anxiety, normal skin color, strong cough, normal level of consciousness, normal oxygen saturation, adequate air movement

2. How will you manage this child's condition initially?

In the conscious child, initial attempts to relieve a severe airway obstruction involve performing abdominal thrusts (Heimlich maneuver).

In the sitting or standing child, kneel on one knee behind the child and place your fist superior to the umbilicus and well below the xiphoid process (subdiaphragmatic region). Place your other hand over your fist and administer abdominal thrusts in an inward-upward direction (**Figure 11-1**). Each thrust should be its own distinct motion, with the intent of removing the obstruction. Avoid applying force to the lower rib cage or sternum as this can cause fractured ribs and internal injury (ie, pneumothorax, liver laceration). Continue administering abdominal thrusts until the child expels the object or loses consciousness.

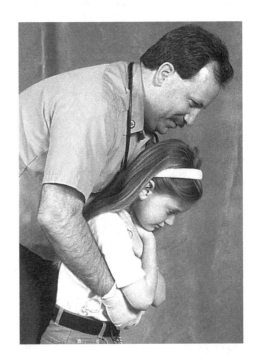

■ **Figure 11-1** Perform abdominal thrusts to treat a severe airway obstruction in a conscious child.

3. What is your next action in the management of this child?

If a child with a severe airway obstruction becomes unconscious, place him or her in a supine position, open the airway with the head tilt–chin lift maneuver, and look in the mouth. If the foreign body is visible, try to remove it with your finger. *Do not perform blind finger sweeps in any unconscious patient with a severe airway obstruction; doing so may force the object further into the pharynx.* If you are unable to visualize a foreign body in the mouth, proceed as follows:

1. **Attempt to ventilate**
   - If the first ventilation does not produce chest rise, reposition the child's head and reattempt to ventilate.

2. **If both ventilations do not produce chest rise, begin chest compressions[1]**
   - If you are by yourself, perform 30 chest compressions
   - If two paramedics are present, perform 15 chest compressions

3. **Open the airway and look in the mouth for a foreign body**

4. **Repeat steps 1 through 3 until the obstruction is removed or you are prepared to perform more advanced techniques**

[1] *In the child (1 year of age to the onset of puberty [12 to 14 years of age]), perform compressions with one or two hands, depending on the size of the child.*

According to the 2005 Emergency Cardiac Care (ECC) guidelines, there is no evidence that abdominal thrusts are superior to chest compressions in relieving a foreign body airway obstruction in unconscious patients. In fact, some studies demonstrated that chest compressions increased intrathoracic pressure as high as or higher than abdominal thrusts.

4. What intervention is indicated now?

If the foreign body is imbedded deep in the soft tissues of the child's airway, the basic life support maneuvers previously discussed may not be successful in relieving the obstruction. If several attempts to relieve an airway obstruction with basic maneuvers are unsuccessful, you should visualize the airway with a laryngoscope (direct laryngoscopy) and attempt to remove the obstruction with Magill forceps. The unique curvature of the Magill forceps allows the paramedic to maneuver them in the airway, and, after visualizing the obstruction, retrieve it from the upper airway (**Figure 11-2**).

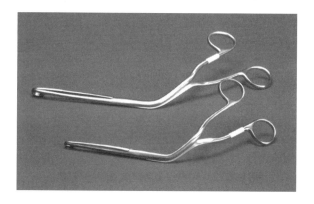

■ **Figure 11-2** Magill forceps have a unique curvature that allows the paramedic to maneuver them in the airway.

To perform laryngoscopy, insert a pediatric-sized straight blade into the child's mouth, advance it, and watch the tip of the blade until the foreign body is visible. Do not advance the blade beyond the vocal cords. If secretions are present in the airway, use suction to improve your laryngoscopic view. Once the foreign body is visualized, insert the Magill forceps into the child's mouth with the tips closed. Grasp the object while maintaining visualization of the airway (**Figure 11-3**).

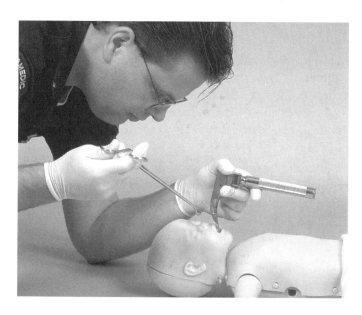

■ **Figure 11-3** Removal of a foreign body with direct laryngoscopy and Magill forceps.

After removing the object, look at the upper airway to make sure it is clear of foreign bodies or debris. Then reassess the child's ventilatory status, suction the airway as needed (no more than 10 seconds in the child), and attempt to ventilate if the child does not resume spontaneous breathing.

If attempts to ventilate are still unsuccessful, attempt to intubate the child. If the object is lodged beyond the vocal cords, it may be necessary to push the object into the right mainstem bronchus, allowing ventilation of the left lung.

If all techniques to remove the obstruction fail (eg, chest compressions, laryngoscopy, intubation), your only other option is to perform a cricothyrotomy. You must be able to secure a patent airway quickly or the child will die. Follow local protocols regarding cricothyrotomy in the child.

5. How will you continue to manage this child's condition?

Although you have successfully removed the child's airway obstruction, he remains apneic. Additionally, his heart rate, cyanosis, and low oxygen saturation indicate significant hypoxemia. Therefore, you must continue positive-pressure ventilations with a bag-valve-mask device and 100% oxygen. Consider inserting an oropharyngeal airway to assist in maintaining a patent airway. In the apneic child with a pulse, ventilations are performed at a rate of 12–20 breaths/min (one breath every 3–5 seconds). Preoxygenate the child sufficiently to cause an increase in his heart rate (> 100 beats/min) and an oxygen saturation as close to 100% as possible. You should then perform endotracheal intubation, on the basis of the following indications:

- **Failure to resume spontaneous respirations following removal of the airway obstruction**
  - It is likely that this child will require prolonged ventilatory support.

- **Nobody to assist you in the back of the ambulance and a lengthy (30 miles) transport to the hospital**
  - When bag-valve-mask ventilations are performed on an apneic patient, cricoid pressure (Sellick maneuver) should be used to minimize the incidence of gastric distention and the associated risk of regurgitation with aspiration. You cannot effectively ventilate the child—or any patient for that matter—*and* perform cricoid pressure by yourself.

Stimulation of the parasympathetic nervous system and bradycardia can occur during intubation; therefore, a cardiac monitor should be applied. Additionally, a pulse oximeter should be utilized prior to, during, and after the intubation attempt in order to monitor the patient's oxygen saturation.

The incidence of vagal-induced bradycardia can be minimized by adequately preoxygenating the child, carefully manipulating the laryngoscope blade in the upper airway, and limiting your intubation attempt to 20 seconds. If bradycardia or a decrease in oxygen saturation below 90% is observed, abort the intubation attempt and reoxygenate the child with a bag-valve-mask device and 100% oxygen until the heart rate and oxygen saturation improve.

You should premedicate children 5 years of age and under with atropine sulfate 0.02 mg/kg (minimum dose of 0.1 mg) prior to intubation in order to prevent vagal-induced bradycardia. Local protocol may require premedication with atropine in children older than 5 years of age.

6. Should you extubate this child? Why or why not?

No! Although the child is becoming restless and agitated, his level of consciousness is not adequate to maintain his own airway. Additionally, his respiratory efforts—albeit spontaneous—are only occasional. Therefore, he is still in need of ventilatory assistance.

There are several risks associated with extubation of emergency patients; therefore, the procedure is rarely performed in the prehospital setting. You must not overestimate the patient's ability to protect his or her own airway. Once the ET tube is removed, there is no guarantee that you will be able to replace it.

Conscious or semiconscious patients are at risk for laryngospasm upon removal of the ET tube, and most patients experience some degree of upper airway swelling due to the trauma of having a tube in their throat. Because this child required laryngoscopy to remove his airway obstruction, you should assume that he is at an even higher risk for extubation-induced laryngospasm.

There is also the ever-present possibility that the child could vomit upon removing the tube. Not only would this pose a threat for aspiration, but it would make reintubation extremely difficult, if not impossible, to perform.

It would be more prudent to sedate this child in order to facilitate his tolerance of the ET tube. **Table 11-5** summarizes the medications, with their pediatric doses, that are commonly used for sedation. Depending on local protocol, other medications may be used to induce sedation.

Table 11-5 Commonly Used Sedative Medications

Midazolam (Versed)
- 0.1-0.2 mg/kg via IV or IM administration
- Maximum single dose of 4 mg

Diazepam (Valium)
- 0.1-0.2 mg/kg via IV administration
- Maximum single dose of 4 mg

Lorazepam (Ativan)
- 0.1 mg/kg via IV or IM administration
- Maximum single dose of 2-4 mg
- Diluted for IV use; undiluted for IM use

Because the child is having spontaneous respiratory effort, you should disconnect the automatic transport ventilator (ATV) and resume assisted ventilation with a bag-valve-mask device and 100% oxygen attached to the ET tube. Most ATVs are used for apneic patients and do not allow the patient to control their own breathing. In intubated patients who resume spontaneous breathing, this will cause increased agitation as they attempt to breathe against the ventilations delivered by the ATV.

Summary

Obstruction of the airway is a dire emergency that requires immediate treatment in order to prevent death. Infants and small children are especially prone to foreign body airway obstructions—most often caused by small toys or objects.

A foreign body airway obstruction should be suspected in an otherwise healthy child without fever who presents with acute coughing, gagging, or increased work of breathing.

Foreign body airway obstructions are classified as being severe or mild. With a severe airway obstruction, the child is not able to cough, speak, or move air. Death will occur soon if the airway obstruction is not immediately removed.

A child with a mild airway obstruction typically presents with anxiety, an effective cough, normal skin color, a normal level of consciousness, and normal oxygen saturation. Treatment for a child with a mild airway obstruction is supportive, and includes encouraging the child to cough, avoiding agitation, providing oxygen as tolerated, and transporting to the hospital.

Because BLS maneuvers are quick to perform and are often all that is needed to remove the airway obstruction, they should be attempted first. However, you should not waste a great deal of time if these simple maneuvers are unsuccessful. In such cases, visualize the airway with a laryngoscope and attempt to remove the obstruction with Magill forceps.

If BLS techniques and laryngoscopy are unsuccessful, a cricothyrotomy may be the child's only chance for survival. Follow local protocol with regard to performing cricothyrotomy in children.

Once the obstruction is removed, reassess the child's airway and breathing status and provide ventilations if spontaneous breathing does not resume or if respiratory effort is inadequate (eg, reduced tidal volume). Consider endotracheal intubation to protect the apneic (or unconscious) child's airway from the threat of aspiration—especially if you are alone in the back of the ambulance with the patient, in which case you will be unable to provide effective bag-valve-mask ventilations and cricoid pressure by yourself.

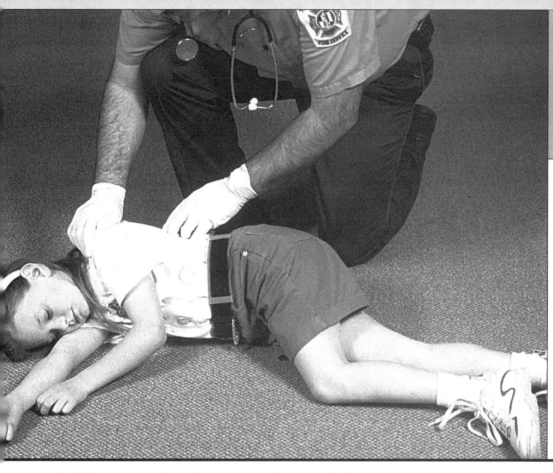

12

10-Year-Old Female Who Is Unresponsive

At 1:20 PM on a Saturday afternoon, you receive a call to a residence at 915 West Alameda Avenue, where a 10-year-old female is reportedly unconscious. You request backup assistance from another paramedic unit and immediately proceed to the scene. Your response time is approximately 7 minutes.

You arrive at the scene at 1:27 PM and are met at the door of the residence by the child's mother. As she escorts you to the child, she explains that her daughter is a diabetic and has recently been ill and running a low-grade fever. As you approach the child, you find her lying on her right side on the floor with a small amount of vomitus near her mouth; she is not moving. The child's mother denies the possibility of trauma and states that she moved her daughter from the couch to the floor. As your partner prepares the oxygen equipment, you perform an initial assessment (**Table 12-1**).

Table 12-1 Initial Assessment

Level of Consciousness	Unconscious and unresponsive
Chief Complaint	Altered mental status/unconscious
Airway and Breathing	Vomitus in the mouth; respirations, rapid and shallow
Circulation	Radial pulse, rapid and weak; skin, warm and moist; no gross bleeding

1. What initial management is indicated for this child?

_____

_____

_____

_____

Your backup paramedic crew arrives at the scene and begins assisting with patient care. One of the paramedics assists your partner in managing the child's airway as the other obtains a blood glucose reading. Because the child is unconscious, you perform a rapid assessment to detect other potentially life-threatening conditions (**Table 12-2**).

Table 12-2 Rapid Assessment

Head	No gross trauma; cranium is stable; pupils, dilated and sluggishly reactive
Neck	Trachea, midline; jugular veins, normal; no cervical spine deformities
Chest	No gross trauma; chest wall movement, symmetrical; breath sounds, clear and equal bilaterally to auscultation
Abdomen and Pelvis	Abdomen, soft and nondistended; pelvis, stable to palpation
Lower Extremities	No gross trauma; pedal pulses, bilaterally present
Upper Extremities	No gross trauma; radial pulses, bilaterally present but weak
Posterior	No gross trauma

The child's blood glucose level is 38 mg/dL. As your partner and the assisting paramedic continue to manage the child's airway, you prepare to initiate an IV line of normal saline. The second assisting paramedic retrieves the stretcher from the ambulance. A concerned neighbor, who saw the ambulances in front of the house, provides emotional support for the child's mother.

2. What are some common causes of hypoglycemia in children?

_____

_____

_____

_____

3. What are the signs and symptoms of hypoglycemia in children?

_____

_____

_____

Your paramedic assistant returns with the ambulance stretcher. The mother tells you that her daughter took her insulin today as prescribed. However, because of her illness, she has not been eating well and has vomited several times. You secure the IV in place and then open the drug kit in preparation for further treatment.

4. What specific therapy is indicated for this child's condition?

_____

_____

_____

Following the appropriate treatment, the child's level of consciousness improves. She begins pushing the bag-valve-mask away from her face, so you apply a nonrebreathing mask at 15 L/min, which she tolerates. A repeat blood glucose assessment reads 95 mg/dL. After obtaining baseline vital signs and a SAMPLE history (**Table 12-3**), the child is placed onto the stretcher, loaded into the ambulance, and transported to the hospital. The mother accompanies her daughter in the ambulance and rides in the front seat.

Table 12-3 Baseline Vital Signs and SAMPLE History

Blood Pressure	98/56 mm Hg
Pulse	120 beats/min, strong and regular
Respirations	24 breaths/min, adequate depth
Oxygen Saturation	99% (on 100% oxygen)
Signs and Symptoms	Hypoglycemia (resolved), unconscious (resolved), recent illness
Allergies	None
Medications	Insulin
Pertinent Past History	Insulin-dependant diabetes
Last Oral Intake	According to the mother, "She last ate 5 hours ago, but vomited shortly thereafter."
Events Leading to Present Illness	Recent illness with fever, poor oral intake, became unconscious on the couch."

En route to the hospital, you administer a 20-mL/kg bolus of normal saline because the child appears to be dehydrated. Her condition continues to improve and she asks you what happened to her. After explaining the series of events to the child, you perform an ongoing assessment (**Table 12-4**) and then call your radio report to the receiving facility, which is 5 minutes away.

Table 12-4 Ongoing Assessment

Level of Consciousness	Conscious and alert to person, place, and time
Airway and Breathing	Airway is patent; respirations, 22 breaths/min with adequate depth
Oxygen Saturation	98% (on 100% oxygen)
Blood Pressure	102/60 mm Hg
Pulse	100 beats/min, strong and regular

You arrive at the emergency department and give your verbal report to the attending physician. After further evaluation in the emergency department, the child was diagnosed with viral gastroenteritis and admitted overnight for observation and fluid rehydration. She was discharged home the following day.

1. What initial management is indicated for this child?

■ **Obtain a patent airway**

First and foremost, you must suction the vomitus from the child's mouth to prevent her from aspirating it. Mortality increases significantly if a patient aspirates vomitus, blood, or secretions into the lungs.

To assist in maintaining airway patency, insert an oropharyngeal or nasopharyngeal airway, depending on the presence or absence of a gag reflex.

■ **Positive-pressure ventilatory assistance**

Rapid, shallow respirations do not produce the amount of tidal volume needed to support adequate minute volume. Decreased minute volume reduces the amount of oxygen and carbon dioxide that is exchanged in the lungs and, ultimately, at the cellular level.

Shallow respirations, which indicate reduced tidal volume, are evidenced by minimal rise of the patient's chest during inhalation. When respirations are both rapid and shallow, the relatively small volume of inhaled air may only make it to the anatomic dead space (trachea and mainstem bronchi) before it is promptly exhaled. This results in hypoxemia and respiratory acidosis due to inadequate oxygen intake and decreased carbon dioxide elimination.

If left untreated, inadequate ventilation will result in metabolic acidosis when the body's cells transition from aerobic to anaerobic metabolism, the byproducts of which are lactic and pyruvic acid.

To restore tidal volume and improve minute volume, assist the child's breathing with a bag-valve-mask device and 100% oxygen. Passive oxygenation devices, such as the nonrebreathing mask, will not deliver oxygen via positive-pressure and are thus ineffective in treating a patient with inadequate ventilation.

A concern when ventilating an unintubated patient is the incidence of gastric distention, which increases the risk of regurgitation with aspiration. This risk is especially high in infants and children, whose stomachs are smaller and can accommodate smaller volumes of air than adults. As air enters the stomach, pressure is applied upward, against the diaphragm, reducing your ability to deliver effective tidal volume with positive-pressure ventilations.

Applying posterior cricoid pressure (Sellick maneuver) minimizes the risks of gastric distention, regurgitation, and aspiration by occluding the esophagus and facilitating airflow into the lungs (**Figure 12-1**).

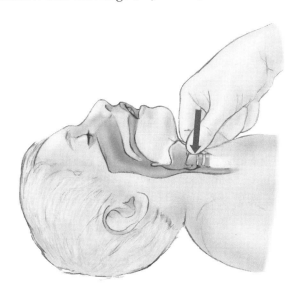

■ **Figure 12-1** Posterior cricoid pressure minimizes the incidence of gastric distention and the associated risk of regurgitation with aspiration by occluding the esophagus, thus facilitating airflow into the lungs.

2. What are some common causes of hypoglycemia in children?

Common causes of hypoglycemia in children are essentially the same as they are in adults (**Table 12-5**). However, children have a greater propensity to develop acute hypoglycemia for several reasons.

Children have inherently limited stores of glycogen, a concentrated form of glucose that is produced by and stored in the liver. When the body requires more glucose, alpha cells in the pancreas secrete glucagon, a protein hormone. When released, glucagon increases blood glucose by facilitating the conversion of glycogen to glucose (glycogenolysis) and stimulating glucose synthesis (gluconeogenesis [production of new glucose]).

During an acute illness, higher than normal levels of glucose are required to fuel the immune response to the illness (ie, fever). In an adult, the body is usually able to accommodate the increased demand for glucose by increasing the process of glycogenolysis. In children, however, the supply of glucose cannot keep up with the increased demand, and their body is quickly depleted of circulating glucose as well as glycogen stores in the liver. To compound the problem, sick children often have poor oral intake or vomiting/diarrhea, which further decreases their ability to increase circulating blood glucose levels. Excessive loss of body water through vomiting or diarrhea may lead to electrolyte derangements; sodium, potassium, and other key electrolytes can be quickly depleted from the child's body.

Table 12-5 Causes of Hypoglycemia in Children
Inadequate oral intake
Severe illness
• Fever
• Vomiting and diarrhea
• Dehydration
Excessive exertion
Insulin imbalance in the diabetic child
• Inadvertent overdose of insulin
• Taking insulin as prescribed but not eating
Intoxication with alcohol or other drugs
• More common in teenagers

The most common scenario for prehospital hypoglycemia is a child with a known history of diabetes who uses too much insulin, exerts him- or herself excessively, or delays a meal.

It is important to note that a patient, especially a child, does not necessarily have to be a diabetic to be predisposed to hypoglycemia. This is especially true if the child is ill and has had minimal or no oral intake. Therefore, you should evaluate any acutely ill-appearing child for hypoglycemia, especially if the child has an abnormal appearance or an altered level of consciousness.

Hypoglycemia (insulin shock) in your 10-year-old patient is likely the result of her acute illness, which has resulted in minimal oral intake, vomiting, and fever. The fact that she took her insulin as prescribed has only lowered her blood sugar further.

3. What are the signs and symptoms of hypoglycemia in children?

The signs and symptoms of hypoglycemia are essentially the same in children as they are in adults. However, hypoglycemia in infants and small children may be hard to detect. They often present with nonspecific signs and symptoms such as irritability, tachypnea, tachycardia, decreased interactiveness, or, according to the caregiver, "not acting right." Measure blood glucose and elicit a history of conditions known to cause hypoglycemia in infants and children (ie, illness, fever, etc.).

Hypoglycemia can be classified as being mild, moderate, or severe (**Table 12-6**). Mild hypoglycemia may cause vague symptoms such as hunger, irritability, and weakness, and signs such as agitation, tachypnea, and tachycardia. Signs of moderate hypoglycemia usually reflect the increasing influence of catecholamine release as the body attempts to compensate for lack of sugar to the tissues. Appearance becomes abnormal and level of consciousness becomes impaired. The signs of severe hypoglycemia are dramatic, and include coma, seizures, and signs of hypoperfusion.

Table 12-6 Signs and Symptoms of Hypoglycemia

Mild
- Hunger
- Irritability
- Weakness
- Agitation
- Tachypnea
- Tachycardia

Moderate
- Anxiety
- Blurred vision
- Abdominal pain
- Headache
- Dizziness
- Diaphoresis
- Pallor
- Tremors
- Confusion

Severe
- Seizures
- Coma
- Hypoperfusion

4. What specific therapy is indicated for this child's condition?

Hypoglycemia is a true medical emergency that, unless treated promptly, may result in seizures, permanent brain damage, or death. Treatment is required when the symptomatic child's blood glucose level falls below 60 mg/dL. After establishing IV or IO access, the following regimens of glucose are given, based on the child's age:

- **Less than 2 years of age**
  - 25% dextrose in water (D_{25}), 2–4 mL/kg
    - Dilute 50% dextrose (D_{50}) to a 1:1 ratio with normal saline to make D_{25}.
- **Older than 2 years of age**
  - 50% dextrose in water (D_{50}), 1–2 mL/kg

Glucose can cause local tissue necrosis if it extravasates; therefore, you should administer it in the largest accessible vein, if possible, and ensure that your IV line is patent.

If IV or IO access is not available, administer 1 mg glucagon via intramuscular (IM) injection. Glucagon will provide a temporary increase in serum glucose by facilitating glycogenolysis; however, it will *only* be effective if there are adequate stores of glycogen in the liver.

Glucagon must be reconstituted (with provided diluent) before administration. Dilute 1 unit (1 mg) of white power (the glucagon) in 1 mL of diluting solution; this will yield a concentration of 1 mg/mL. Do not mix glucagon with normal saline.

Not all EMS systems carry glucagon on their ambulance; therefore, if initial attempts to obtain IV or IO access are unsuccessful, continue oxygen therapy (or assisted ventilation) and immediately transport the hypoglycemic child to the hospital, with continued attempts to obtain venous access en route.

In infants and children, thermal management is an important part of managing hypoglycemia. Without adequate blood glucose, energy production is reduced and thus the ability to maintain body temperature.

Summary

Hypoglycemia, defined as an abnormally low (< 60 mg/dL) level of serum glucose, is a common complication associated with diabetes. However, it can occur in nondiabetic patients as well—especially infants and children, who have limited amounts of glycogen that can be rapidly depleted during a severe illness.

Suspect and evaluate for hypoglycemia in any ill-appearing child, especially if their appearance is abnormal or their mental status is altered. If left untreated, hypoglycemia can result in seizures, permanent brain damage, or even death. To avoid this potential disaster, a rapid evaluation and prompt treatment is required.

Treatment for hypoglycemia begins by ensuring a patent airway and adequate breathing and administering 100% oxygen or assisted ventilation as needed. Establish an IV line or insert an IO cannula and administer 1–2 mL/kg of D_{50} in children older than 2 years of age (2–4 mL/kg of D_{25} in children less than 2 years of age). If IV or IO access is not possible, administer 1 mg of glucagon IM, if available. Further management consists of maintaining the ABCs, preserving body temperature, and promptly transporting the child to the hospital.

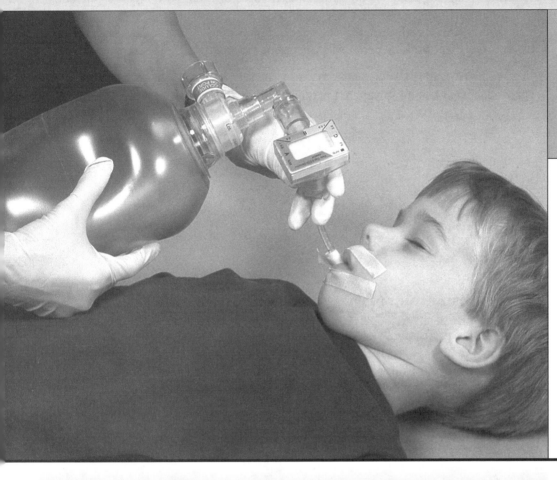

13

5-Year-Old Male Who Is Not Breathing

At 2:35 PM, you receive a call to 211 East Rosewood for a "child not breathing." You request first responder assistance and immediately proceed to the scene, with a response time of approximately 8 minutes.

Upon your arrival, first responders are performing bag-valve-mask ventilations on the child, a 5-year-old boy. As your partner opens the jump kit, you proceed with an initial assessment of the child (**Table 13-1**). The child's mother tells you that her son was taking a nap in his room. When she went to wake him up, she discovered that he was not breathing. There are no suspicious findings in the environment in which the child was found.

Table 13-1 Initial Assessment

Level of Consciousness	Unconscious and unresponsive
Chief Complaint	Unconscious and not breathing
Airway and Breathing	Airway is patent; respirations, absent
Circulation	Radial pulse, slow and weak; capillary refill time, 3 seconds; skin, pale and cool; no gross bleeding

A rapid assessment of the child reveals no gross trauma or bleeding. Your partner inserts an oropharyngeal airway, and, while a first responder applies cricoid pressure, he continues bag-valve-mask ventilations with 100% oxygen. However, despite effective ventilations, the child's heart rate remains slow. You attach a cardiac monitor, which reveals sinus bradycardia at 40 beats/min. The child's mother states that her son has no medical problems and was fine earlier in the day.

1. What additional basic life support is indicated for this child?

The appropriate basic life support is being performed on the child, who remains apneic and bradycardic. You make several attempts to start an IV line without success. As you are preparing to obtain intraosseous access, you ask the child's mother if there is any possibility that the child could have ingested any medications or chemicals. The mother goes to investigate under the sink and in the medicine cabinet.

2. What are the indications for intraosseous access in children? How is the procedure performed?

Intraosseous access has been successfully established and blood glucose analysis reveals a reading of 104 mg/dL. Chest compressions and bag-valve-mask ventilations are continued at the appropriate rate. You glance at the cardiac monitor and note that the child's heart rate is 50 beats/min, which corresponds with his radial pulse. After premedicating the child with 0.02 mg/kg of atropine, your partner successfully performs endotracheal intubation. Correct placement of the ET tube is confirmed by auscultation and capnography.

3. What initial drug is used to treat refractory bradycardia in children?

You administer the appropriate medication, after which you note an increase in the child's heart rate to 90 beats/min. Chest compressions are stopped but ventilations are continued at the appropriate rate. The child's mother returns with an open bottle of her husband's clonazepam (Klonopin), which she found on the floor in the bathroom. The prescription was filled 4 days prior with 30 1-mg tablets; however, there are only 5 tablets remaining. You assess the child's pupils and note that they are equal, dilated, and sluggishly reactive.

4. Would naloxone be effective in treating this ingestion? Why or why not?

A first responder retrieves the stretcher from the ambulance and you prepare to transport the child to a hospital located 20 miles away. The child is loaded into the ambulance, where you quickly obtain baseline vital signs and a SAMPLE history (**Table 13-2**). The child's mother provides you with the necessary information.

Table 13-2 Baseline Vital Signs and SAMPLE History

Blood Pressure	86/56 mm Hg
Pulse	110 beats/min and regular; stronger than before
Respirations	Intubated and ventilated with 100% oxygen at 15 breaths/min
Oxygen Saturation	98% (with ventilations and 100% oxygen)
ECG	Normal sinus rhythm
Signs and Symptoms	Apnea, bradycardia (resolved)
Allergies	None
Medications	None
Pertinent Past History	None
Last Oral Intake	A sandwich approximately 3 hours ago
Events Leading to Present Illness	"I guess he got into the medicine cabinet when I wasn't looking. When I went to wake him up, I noticed that he wasn't breathing. I started mouth-to-mouth on him until the responders arrived."
Child's Weight	According to mother, about 40 pounds (18 kg)

Because your partner's assistance is needed in the back of the ambulance for appropriate patient care, you ask a first responder to drive the ambulance to the hospital. The child's mother tells you that she will follow you in her car. You advise her to drive safely, and that you will meet her at the emergency department.

5. What actions should you perform while en route to the hospital?

_____

_____

_____

_____

The child's heart rate remains stable throughout transport; however, he remains apneic. Your partner continues ventilations and monitors correct ET tube placement with digital capnometry. You perform an ongoing assessment (**Table 13-3**), then call your radio report to the receiving facility.

Table 13-3 Ongoing Assessment

Level of Consciousness	Unconscious and unresponsive
Airway and Breathing	Intubated; ventilated with 100% oxygen at 15 breaths/min
Oxygen Saturation	98% (with ventilations and 100% oxygen)
Blood Pressure	90/60 mm Hg
Pulse	118 beats/min, strong and regular
Capillary Refill Time	2 seconds
Capnometry	Reads 38 mm Hg
ECG	Normal sinus rhythm

You arrive at the hospital after an uneventful transport and give your verbal report to the attending physician. A toxicology screen of the child's blood reveals benzodiazepines, but no other CNS depressants or illicit substances. After further assessment and treatment in the emergency department, the child is placed on a mechanical ventilator and admitted to the pediatric ICU. He later resumed spontaneous respirations, was weaned off the ventilator and extubated, and was discharged home. The physician educates the child's mother with regard to the safekeeping of medications in the home.

1. What additional basic life support is indicated for this child?

Not only is this child apneic, he is bradycardic as well. Bradycardia in children is an ominous sign and is most often the result of severe hypoxemia. Although a primary respiratory event is the most common precursor to hypoxia in children, this child's mother has confirmed the absence of any previous illnesses. Further assessment will therefore be required in order to determine the underlying etiology of his condition. In a sick child, bradycardia indicates impending cardiopulmonary arrest, which has a significantly high mortality rate. Therefore, the treatment of bradycardia in any symptomatic child—breathing or not—focuses on ensuring a patent airway and supporting oxygenation, ventilation, and perfusion. In the child, symptomatic bradycardia is characterized by poor systemic perfusion (eg, delayed capillary refill, weak or absent peripheral pulses, hypotension), respiratory difficulty, or an altered level of consciousness.

If, despite adequate positive-pressure ventilations with 100% oxygen, the child's heart rate remains below 60 beats/min, further BLS includes initiating chest compressions.

In a child (1 year of age to puberty [12 to 14 years of age]), compress the lower half of the sternum—avoiding the xiphoid process and ribs—with the heel of one *or* two hands, depending on the size of the child. Compressions should be delivered at a depth that is equal to one half to one third the anterior-posterior depth of the chest. Ensure that you allow full recoil of the chest in between compressions.

For one-rescuer child CPR, perform a compression-to-ventilation ratio of 30:2 (**Figure 13-1**). Two-rescuer child CPR is performed at a compression-to-ventilation ratio of 15:2. In the nonintubated child, ventilations and chest compressions should be synchronous; coordinate compressions with ventilations, pausing compressions to deliver the ventilations.

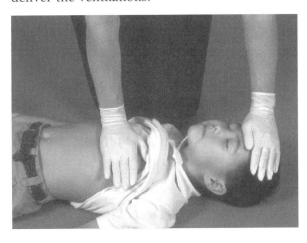

■ **Figure 13-1** In a child, compress the lower half of the sternum, avoiding the xiphoid process and ribs, with the heel of one or two hands. Perform compressions and ventilations synchronously until the child is intubated.

2. What are the indications for intraosseous access in children? How is the procedure performed?

When peripheral perfusion in a child is decreased, IV access is often difficult to obtain, especially in infants and small children. Veins that may have otherwise been visible when cardiac output was adequate tend to collapse.

Intraosseous (IO) access is indicated in the severely ill or injured child when IV access is unsuccessful. Most texts and clinicians agree that if IV access is unsuccessful after 90 seconds *or* three attempts, the paramedic should proceed with IO access in order to obtain emergent vascular access. Some protocols, however, state that the paramedic should proceed immediately with IO access if IV access is anticipated to be difficult or impossible to obtain, especially if the child is critically ill or injured.

IO access allows for the administration of drugs, volume expanders (eg, normal saline, lactated Ringer's solution), and blood products directly into the medullary cavity of the bone, which is highly vascularized. From the medullary cavity, blood drains into the central venous canal and then directly into the central circulation. Most IO-administered medications are comparable to IV administration with regard to onset of action and achievement of therapeutic levels.

IO access requires a special type of catheter (**Figure 13-2**), which is a 14- to 16-gauge stainless steel needle with a stylet (trochar) through its center.

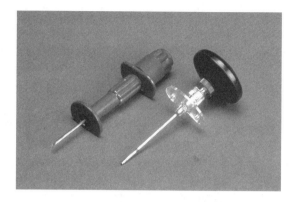

■ **Figure 13-2** An IO catheter is a 14- to 16-gauge stainless steel needle with a stylet (trochar) through its center.

There are several possible sites that are suitable for IO access, such as the femur or distal tibia; however, the preferred location is the proximal tibia. First, locate the tibial tuberosity, which is the bony protuberance just inferior to the knee. Then, palpate the flat proximal tibia, which usually can be found 1 to 2 finger widths medial to the tibial tuberosity, depending on the size of the child.

Cleanse the site appropriately. Then, while pulling the skin over the insertion site tight, insert the IO needle through the skin, directing it away from the epiphysis—the growth plate of the bone. Pierce the cortex (outer layer of the bone) with a firm, twisting motion. A "pop" or sudden release in pressure may be felt as the needle passes through the bony cortex and into the medullary cavity (**Figure 13-3**). Avoid too much force when inserting the needle, as this may cause the needle to penetrate all the way through the bone and into the soft tissues beyond. It is important to insert the IO needle at a 90° angle in order to avoid missing the bone.

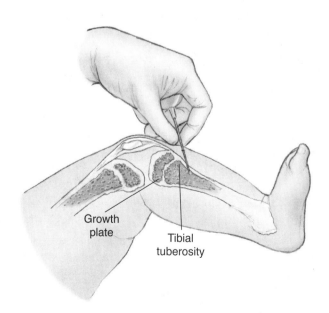

■ **Figure 13-3**
An IO needle inserted into the medullary cavity.

Once the needle has entered the medullary cavity, remove the stylet and aspirate for marrow contents. Bone marrow aspirate can be used for blood glucose testing if needed. Sometimes, however, marrow cannot be aspirated; this is not necessarily an indication that IO placement was unsuccessful.

Correct placement is confirmed when you can infuse 10 mL of normal saline with little resistance and when the needle is stable (does not flop around) in the bone. Attach the IV line to the hub of the IO catheter; use of extension tubing and a stopcock valve is optional. Infuse fluids or drugs directly into the intraosseous space (**Figure 13-4**).

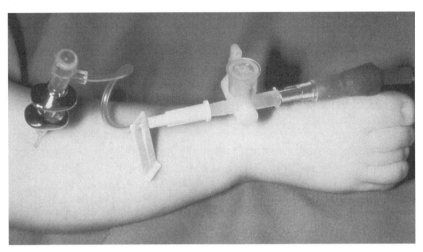

■ **Figure 13-4** A correctly placed IO needle with an IV line attached.

Secure the IO needle in place with bulky dressing and tape—just as you would stabilize an impaled object in place. Monitor the calf to ensure that there is no swelling, which would indicate leakage of fluid secondary to through-and-through penetration of the bone. The indications, contraindications, and potential complications of IO access are summarized in **Table 13-4**.

Table 13-4 Indications, Contraindications, and Potential Complications of IO Access

Indications
- IV access cannot be obtained within 3 attempts or 90 seconds.
- IV access is anticipated to be difficult or impossible.
- The child is critically ill or injured.

Contraindications
- Absolute Contraindications
  - A patent IV line is established.
  - Fracture of the bone considered for access
  - Recent IO cannulation of the bone considered for access
  - Known osteogenesis imperfecta or osteopetrosis
    - Congenital bone diseases
  - Known osteoporosis
    - Extremely rare in children
- Relative Contraindications
  - Deep burns
  - Cellulitis
  - Infectious process at the site of insertion

(Continued)

Potential Complications
- Compartment syndrome
  - Can occur if extravasation of fluid is undetected
- Osteomyelitis
  - Infection of the bone and adjacent muscle
  - Risk is minimal if the insertion site is appropriately cleansed and the IO cannula is removed within 24 hours.
- Growth plate injury
  - Can be avoided by identifying the correct anatomic landmark and using proper technique
- Fracture
  - May occur if the extremity is not properly stabilized or if the IO needle is inserted in the incorrect site where the bone is weaker

The primary technical problem with IO access is successfully piercing the bony cortex in older children. The bones in neonates, infants, and small children are usually soft and the intraosseous space is relatively large, so IO needle insertion is easier in children in these younger age groups.

Although IO access is easy, quick, and relatively safe, it is extremely painful in the conscious child and is therefore only practical if the child is unconscious or otherwise critically ill or injured.

3. What initial drug is used to treat refractory bradycardia in children?

Most clinically significant bradycardic rhythms in children are the result of hypoxemia; therefore, the need for immediate support of oxygenation and ventilation deserves re-emphasis.

However, if despite effective oxygenation and ventilation and chest compressions, the child remains symptomatically bradycardic (heart rate < 60 beats/min), epinephrine is the initial pharmacological agent of choice, as recommended by the American Academy of Pediatrics. Epinephrine is a sympathomimetic agent that possesses both alpha- and beta-adrenergic properties. The beta-adrenergic effects increase heart rate (chronotropy) and myocardial contractility (inotropy), while the alpha-adrenergic effects cause vasoconstriction and increase blood pressure.

Epinephrine, like all catecholamines, may cause an increase in myocardial oxygen demand and consumption. Additionally, the effectiveness of catecholamines may be reduced by hypoxemia and acidosis. Therefore, concomitant support of oxygenation, ventilation, and perfusion (with chest compressions) is essential.

The dose of epinephrine in children depends on the route of administration:

- **IV or IO administration**
  - 0.01 mg/kg (0.1 mL/kg) of a 1:10,000 solution
    - Repeat every 3 to 5 minutes at the same dose.
- **Endotracheal administration**
  - 0.1 mg/kg (0.1 mL/kg) of a 1:1,000 solution
    - Repeat every 3 to 5 minutes at the same dose.

Atropine, a parasympatholytic agent, increases the rate of SA node discharge and enhances conduction through the AV node, making it a useful drug in treating vagal-induced bradycardia. Unless associated with intubation, primary vagal-induced bradycardia in children is an uncommon event. However, if increased vagal tone or primary

AV block is the suspected cause of the bradycardia, atropine, in the following dosing regimen, should precede the administration of epinephrine:

- **0.02 mg/kg via rapid IV or IO administration**
  - Minimum single dose: 0.1 mg
    - Maximum single dose in a child is 0.5 mg; 1 mg in an adolescent.
    - Maximum total dose in a child is 1 mg; 2 mg in an adolescent.
  - May be repeated once in 3 to 5 minutes

Transcutaneous cardiac pacing (TCP) should be considered for bradycardia that is refractory to oxygenation and ventilation, chest compressions, epinephrine, and atropine.

4. Would naloxone be effective in treating this ingestion? Why or why not?

Clonazepam (Klonopin), a CNS depressant, is a benzodiazepine sedative-hypnotic drug commonly prescribed for the treatment of conditions such as anxiety, insomnia, and seizures. Klonopin is *not* a narcotic (opiate); therefore, naloxone (Narcan), which binds to opiate receptor sites in the body and antagonizes (blocks) the effects of narcotics, would be ineffective in reversing the CNS depressant effects associated with this child's ingestion.

Based on when the prescription was refilled and the number of pills remaining in the bottle, this 5-year-old child has ingested 21 mg of Klonopin. Additionally, Klonopin, relative to other benzodiazepines (**Table 13-5**), has a longer duration of action. These factors clearly explain his unconsciousness, apnea, and bradycardia.

Table 13-5 Commonly Prescribed Benzodiazepines

Short-acting
- Temazepam (Restoril)
- Triazolam (Halcion)
- Estazolam (ProSom)
- Flurazepam (Dalmane)

Long-acting
- Clonazepam (Klonopin)
- Alprazolam (Xanax)
- Chlordiazepoxide (Librium)
- Diazepam (Valium)
- Clorazepate (Tranxene)
- Halazepam (Paxipam)
- Lorazepam (Ativan)

Flumazenil (Romazicon), an imidazobenzodiazepine, is a benzodiazepine antagonist that blocks the central effects of agents that act via the benzodiazepine receptor by competitive inhibition.

Flumazenil has been shown to successfully reverse benzodiazepine-induced sedation in adults; however, it is not as effective in reversing hypoventilation. Furthermore, many EMS systems do not carry flumazenil. It is, however, used in children in the hospital setting for acute benzodiazepine overdose. When treating a child with benzodiazepine-induced CNS depression, the most important prehospital treatment is to support oxygenation, ventilation, and perfusion. If prolonged ventilatory support will be required, intubate the child to prevent gastric distention and aspiration if regurgitation occurs. Obtain venous or IO access and administer epinephrine for bradycardia that is refractory to chest compressions.

In some cases, children will ingest several different medications, each of which possesses different physiologic effects. If concomitant narcotic ingestion is suspected or cannot be ruled out, administer naloxone (IV, IM, or ET) in the following dose:

- ≤ 5 years old or ≤ 20 kg: 0.1 mg/kg
- ≥ 5 years old or ≥ 20 kg: 2 mg

5. What actions should you perform while en route to the hospital?

Considering that a reversal agent for benzodiazepine toxicity is usually not available in the prehospital setting, you have performed all the necessary actions to support this child's ventilatory and circulatory functions. Therefore, further management consists of continuing positive-pressure ventilations and close, continuous monitoring.

A crucial aspect in managing the ill or injured child is to perform *frequent* cardiopulmonary assessments. Monitor blood pressure, heart rate, and perfusion, and be prepared to intervene immediately if the child's condition deteriorates. If the intubated child's condition deteriorates (eg, bradycardia, low oxygen saturation), consider mechanical problems with oxygenation and ventilation. The DOPE mnemonic (**Table 13-6**) is a useful tool to help troubleshoot potential causes of acute deterioration in the intubated child.

Table 13-6 Troubleshooting Acute Deterioration with the DOPE Mnemonic

Dislodgement of the ET tube
- Inadvertent extubation
  - Lack of chest rise during ventilations
  - Poor or absent air movement on auscultation
  - $ETCO_2$ monitor/detector reads no CO_2 or no color change.
    - Immediately extubate; ventilate with a bag-valve-mask device and 100% oxygen; consider reintubation
- Mainstem bronchus intubation
  - Asymmetric breath sounds
  - Asymmetric chest rise
    - *Slowly* withdraw the tube—while ventilating and auscultating—until breath sounds are equal bilaterally and chest rise is symmetrical.

Obstruction of the ET tube with secretions
- Decreased chest rise
- Decreased breath sounds bilaterally
- Increased resistance when ventilating
  - Perform tracheobronchial suctioning.
  - Extubate and ventilate with a bag-valve-mask device and 100% oxygen if no improvement following tracheobronchial suctioning; consider reintubation.

Pneumothorax (spontaneous or induced)
- Asymmetric chest rise
- Asymmetric breath sounds
- Jugular venous distention[1]
- Tracheal deviation[1]
  - Perform needle thoracentesis (chest decompression) on the side without breath sounds.

Equipment
- Oxygen tubing disconnected
- Oxygen tank empty
- Bag-valve-mask device is defective (eg, torn reservoir, damaged bag)
  - Check equipment from "patient-to-tank."

[1]Not easily assessed in infants and small children

If the child's condition deteriorates and technical problems are ruled out (eg, DOPE), be prepared to initiate chest compressions and administer additional epinephrine boluses. If hypotension develops, assess the child's volume status and consider crystalloid fluid boluses at 20 mL/kg. If hypotension persists, consider an epinephrine or dopamine infusion, titrated to improve perfusion:

- Epinephrine 0.1 to 1 µg/kg/min
- Dopamine 2 to 20 µg/kg/min

Summary

Toxic exposures are a common pediatric complaint in the prehospital setting. Approximately 70% of all toxic exposures occur in children. Eighty percent of childhood poisonings occur in children under 5 years of age. Iron is the leading cause of childhood poisoning deaths, followed by tricyclic antidepressants.

Initial management for a child with a suspected toxic ingestion involves establishing a patent airway and ensuring adequate oxygenation and ventilation. Attempt to ascertain what and how much was ingested and approximately how long ago the ingestion occurred. Contact medical control or the poison control center as dictated by local protocol. Approximating the child's weight in kilograms is important for purposes of administering medications and any antidotes or reversal agents, if available.

There are a host of CNS depressant drugs prescribed for a variety of conditions (eg, anxiety, insomnia, seizures). Such medications include benzodiazepines, narcotics, and barbiturates. Although the physiologic effects of these CNS depressants are similar when taken in excess (eg, decreased LOC, hypoventilation, bradycardia, hypotension), their mechanisms of action are different.

Although generally considered less potent than narcotics, benzodiazepines can cause significant CNS depression when taken in excess, especially in children.

If left untreated, drug-induced CNS depression will result in significant hypoxemia, acidosis, and eventual cardiopulmonary arrest.

Because flumazenil (Romazicon), a benzodiazepine antagonist, is an uncommon prehospital drug, management is aimed at supporting adequate oxygenation, ventilation, and perfusion. Protect the child's airway with an ET tube and establish IV or IO access. If narcotic ingestion is suspected or cannot be ruled out, administer naloxone. If, despite effective oxygenation and ventilation, the child remains symptomatically bradycardic (heart rate < 60 beats/min), chest compressions should be initiated. The initial drug of choice for symptomatic bradycardia in children is epinephrine, which is used to increase heart rate and blood pressure.

Atropine should be administered for epinephrine-refractory bradycardia or if the bradycardia is thought to be vagal-induced or associated with a primary AV block. Consider transcutaneous pacing for children whose bradycardia is refractory to epinephrine and atropine.

Further management consists of prompt transport to the emergency department with continuous monitoring of heart rate, blood pressure, and perfusion en route. Follow local protocols and/or contact medical control as needed for guidance.

A major role of the paramedic is to serve as an advocate for illness and injury prevention. Many pediatric toxic ingestions can be prevented if the parents or caregivers ensure that all medications and toxic chemicals are locked up or stored in a location that is inaccessible to children.

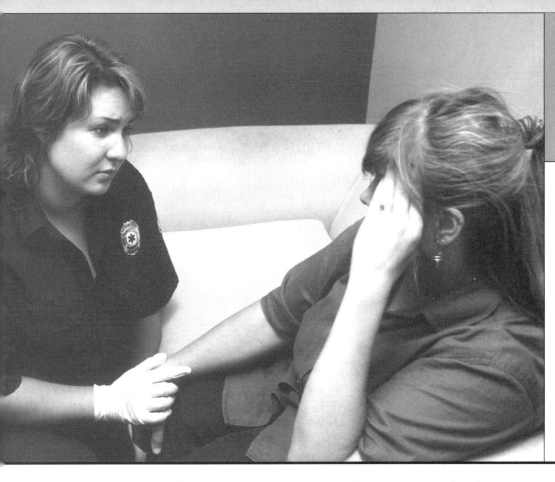

14

2-Month-Old Male with Suspected SIDS

At 7:20 AM on a wintry Saturday morning, you are dispatched to a residence at 655 West Highland Street for an unconscious infant who is not breathing. A first responder unit, located less than a mile from the scene, is dispatched. You and your partner proceed to the scene, with a response time of approximately 9 minutes. While en route, the first responder unit radios you that CPR is in progress. Because of the nature of the call, law enforcement was dispatched with you.

You arrive at the scene at 7:29 AM, enter the residence, and find a first responder performing one-person CPR on the infant, a 2-month-old male. You ask the first responder to stop CPR as you perform an initial assessment (**Table 14-1**). The infant's parents are standing in the corner in disbelief. The mother tells you that she found the baby lying facedown in the crib.

Table 14-1 Initial Assessment

Level of Consciousness	Unconscious and unresponsive
Chief Complaint	Pulseless and apneic
Airway and Breathing	Small amount of blood-tinged fluid in the mouth; respirations, absent
Circulation	No palpable pulse; skin, cold to the touch and pale; dependent mottling; no gross bleeding

1. On the basis of your initial assessment findings, how will you proceed with the management of this situation?

The infant's mother tells you that she fed him at approximately 3:00 AM and that he appeared fine at that time. She further states that he has had no recent illnesses and takes no medications. He was, however, born at 34 weeks' gestation. You and your partner suspect that this is a case of sudden infant death syndrome.

2. What is sudden infant death syndrome?

3. What are some effective ways of communicating with the parents regarding the unexpected death of their child?

_____

_____

_____

_____

After consulting with medical control, you explain to the infant's parents that their son has likely been dead for a prolonged period of time and that resuscitative efforts will not change the outcome. The mother, who is obviously distraught, is being comforted by her husband. After you further explain the situation and answer the parent's questions, they mutually agree that resuscitative efforts should not be attempted.

4. What information should you obtain from the scene and the parents?

_____

_____

_____

_____

The mother asks you if she can hold her baby; you comply with her request. As your partner is offering comfort and support to the parents, a police officer arrives at the scene. You apprise the officer of the situation and your findings. Your local protocols require you to remain at the scene of a suspected SIDS death until the funeral director arrives. The father asks you if there was anything they could have done to prevent this. You advise him that this situation could not have been predicted, nor prevented.

5. How can the prehospital professional help reduce the incidence of SIDS?

_____

_____

_____

_____

You continue to provide emotional support to the infant's parents. The funeral director arrives and transports the infant to the medical examiner's office. Following a thorough investigation, the medical examiner determines that SIDS was indeed the cause of the infant's death.

6. What are some healthy practices for the EMS provider following the sudden death of a child?

14

1. On the basis of your initial assessment findings, how will you proceed with the management of this situation?

Although there are other causes of cardiopulmonary arrest in infants in this age group, sudden infant death syndrome (SIDS) is the most common. Nonetheless, the paramedic's initial actions when SIDS is suspected must always be the assessment and treatment of the baby. Immediately begin resuscitative efforts, following standard or locally established protocols, unless the infant meets your local EMS system's criteria for obvious death.

There is evidence that this infant has been dead for a prolonged period of time (ie, cool, pale skin, dependent mottling [lividity]). In most SIDS cases, obvious signs of death will be present (**Table 14-2**); therefore, resuscitative efforts are typically not indicated. The parents, after being apprised of the situation and expected outcome, will usually permit you to withhold or cease resuscitative efforts. If, however, this is not the case, continue CPR and discuss the futility of attempted resuscitation with the parents. Follow local protocol or contact medical control as needed with regard to the management of a suspected SIDS case.

Table 14-2 Signs of Obvious Death

Dependent Lividity (Livor Mortis)
- Settling of the blood in the lower (dependent) portion of the body, causing a purplish-red discoloration of the skin
- Lividity doesn't appear where the body is in contact with something. Thus, a body lying on its back will show lividity in the small of the back and the neck, but not in parts of the body directly in contact with a surface (ie, ground, crib).

Cold Skin (Algor Mortis)
- Reduction in body temperature following death. This is generally a steady decline until matching ambient temperature, although external factors can have a significant influence on how quickly body temperature falls.

Stiffening of the Joints of the Body (Rigor Mortis)
- Can occur as quickly as 3 hours' postmortem in infants

2. What is sudden infant death syndrome?

Sudden infant death syndrome (SIDS) is the unexpected death of an otherwise healthy infant. In 1989, the National Institute of Child Health and Human Development (NICHD) revised the definition of SIDS as follows: "The sudden and unexpected death of an infant under one year of age, which remains unexplained after a thorough post-mortem evaluation, including performance of a complete autopsy, examination of the death scene, and review of the clinical history."

SIDS is the leading cause of death in infants between 1 month and 1 year of age; it is rare during the first month of life. There are approximately 3,000 SIDS cases per year in the United States. Approximately 90% to 95% of all SIDS deaths occur in infants less than 6 months of age, with a peak incidence in infants between 2 and 4 months of age. Of all SIDS cases, 60% to 70% occur in males, most frequently during the winter months. African American and Native American infants are two to three times more likely to die from SIDS than infants in other ethnic groups.

In approximately 5% of suspected SIDS cases, the medical examiner can identify a specific condition as the cause of death. Such conditions include injury, congenital birth defects, infection, and metabolic disorders. SIDS is a recognized medical disorder; however, its diagnosis can only be made by process of elimination.

The history given to EMS personnel is typically that of a healthy infant between 1 and 6 months of age who was put to bed shortly after a feeding and was subsequently found dead, usually several hours later. Occasionally, a mild upper respiratory infection (ie, cough, runny nose) will be reported prior to the death. The parents or caregivers may have checked on the infant periodically and found nothing out of the ordinary (ie, sounds of a struggle). **Table 14-3** lists the common clinical presentation of SIDS; the signs may differ depending on how long the infant has been dead. In some SIDS cases, however, none of these signs is present.

Table 14-3 Clinical Presentation of SIDS

Algor mortis
Livor mortis
Rigor mortis
Frothy or blood-tinged fluid in the mouth and nose
Normal hydration and nutrition
Vomitus (uncommon)

SIDS cannot be diagnosed in the field by EMS personnel or in the emergency department by a physician. Only after a thorough postmortem examination, to include an autopsy, information about the scene, and the infant's medical history, can a medical examiner determine the cause of death.

3. What are some effective ways of communicating with the parents regarding the unexpected death of their child?

The EMS provider's emotional support of the parents or caregivers is extremely important. Ideally, there should be enough help at the scene to ensure that the parents are appropriately apprised of the situation and are provided the necessary emotional support.

Express condolences to the parents or caregivers and assure them that it is routine to investigate all sudden deaths.

Your skill and sensitivity will set the tone for the parent's or caregiver's interactions with other officials and professionals who will subsequently become involved. Do not attempt to control parent/caregiver reactions during this tragic and emotionally trying time. Ask if there is someone that the parents or caregivers would like you to contact (ie, other family members, neighbor, clergy).

When communicating the infant's death to the parents or caregivers, you should be clear that the infant is dead; do not attempt to relay this information using obscure language or terms, such as "your child has left us" or "he or she has gone to a better place." Avoid unnecessary remarks intended to comfort the parents or caregivers, such as "You can always have other children," "I know how you feel," or "You will get over this in time."

Table 14-4 suggests specific ways to communicate with parents or caregivers when there is an unexpected death of a child.

When responding to a call involving a sudden infant death, you will likely encounter parents/caregivers who have intense and emotionally traumatic reactions to the infant's death. It is important to respect these reactions and feelings.

When confronted with such a sudden and traumatic loss, some parents and caregivers will become angry or even hysterical. Some parents or caregivers may blame themselves; others may withdraw, with no visible response. Denial is a common reaction to the sudden, unexpected death of a child.

Table 14-4 Communicating about an Unexpected Death of a Child

Use the infant's name.
Show empathy and express condolences.
Never project a hostile or angry attitude.
Use a calm and direct voice.
Be clear with instructions and answers to questions.
Provide explanations to the parents/caregivers about treatment and transport.
Repeat statements when necessary.
Reassure parents/caregivers that there was nothing they could have done to prevent this.
If transporting the infant to the emergency department, allow the parent/caregiver to accompany the infant if they so wish.

It is crucial that you remain calm, nonjudgmental, and patient. Parents or caregivers may repeat the same question or questions. Try to explain information regarding the situation in terms that the parent or caregiver can understand.

It is also important to recognize that the parents and family, as well as other caregivers, may have cultural beliefs, values, and practices related to death. The infant's family may have various rituals related to their religious or cultural background that they will want to observe; you must be respectful of this.

4. What information should you obtain from the scene and the parents?

Some protocols require prehospital care providers to transport the dead infant to the hospital, while others require you to remain at the scene until the medical examiner or funeral director arrives.

In many cases, the medical examiner will not be at the death scene. Therefore, he or she will rely on documentation from EMS and law enforcement personnel to help determine the cause of death. Although law enforcement officials may conduct the formal investigation, the prehospital care provider's information about the scene and the infant's history is valuable.

Gathering of information begins when you arrive at the scene and conduct your scene size-up. You should note your findings carefully as these are often important pieces of information for the medical examiner and other personnel who will review the entire case.

Note the location of the infant upon your arrival at the scene (ie, in the crib or bed, on the floor). If the infant was moved prior to your arrival, investigate the location where the death occurred and document whether or not the infant was in his or her own crib. When examining the infant's crib, note the type of sleeping surface (ie, firm, soft) and the type of covering blankets (ie, soft, thick).

If the infant was not moved from the crib, determine if the crib was shared by another sibling. Note whether or not the blanket was over the infant's face at the time of discovery. Document the sleeping position when the infant was placed to sleep and when he or she was discovered. Check for the presence of other objects in the area where the infant was found, especially pillows or other soft or bulky items. Note any unusual conditions such as an excessively high room temperature, strange odors, or the presence of any drugs (illicit and prescription) or drug paraphernalia.

When assessing the infant, look for clues that may indicate potential child maltreatment. These include, among others, visible signs of injury (ie, bruises, cuts, burns) or a malnourished appearance.

At the scene, you should ask questions regarding the circumstances of the death and the infant's medical history. Refrain from asking judgmental or leading questions; open-ended, precise questions are most effective. Ask the infant's name at the beginning of the interview and use his or her first name throughout the discussion. **Table 14-5** lists examples of key questions to ask the parents or caregiver.

Table 14-5 Key Questions in the Focused History of a SIDS Case
Can you tell me what happened?
Where was the infant found?
Who discovered the infant?
What did you do when you discovered the infant?
Has the infant been moved? If so, by whom?
What time was the infant last seen alive?
Had the infant been ill recently?
Was the infant a term baby or premature?
Was the infant taking any medications? If so, what for?

Completely and accurately document all findings of the scene size-up, history, patient assessment, and treatment on the patient care form. Document only factual information; *do not document your opinion or other nonfactual information.* Documenting your observations may be very difficult if you are tending to the infant while providing emotional support to the parents or caregivers. Also, depending on your local protocol, the death scene documentation protocol may be lengthy. If possible, you should assign one person—perhaps a first responder or other official—to document your factual findings as you report them.

5. How can the prehospital professional help reduce the incidence of SIDS?

Although a number of theories exist regarding the etiology of SIDS, its cause remains unknown. Unfortunately, SIDS cannot be predicted or prevented; however, a number of risk factors have been identified (**Table 14-6**). As a prehospital professional, your active role in a community education program may help reduce the incidence of SIDS.

Table 14-6 Risk Factors for SIDS
Formula feeding (possible risk factor)
Prematurity or low birth weight
Young maternal age
Lack of prenatal care
Prone sleeping position • Side-sleeping to a lesser extent
Soft sleeping surfaces
Soft objects in the crib (ie, pillows) • Traps air or gases in the baby's sleeping area
Soft, bulky blankets or comforters
Tobacco smoke exposure • Especially during pregnancy, but after birth as well

The "Back to Sleep" campaign is based on the American Academy of Pediatrics' (AAP) recommendation made in 1992 to place infants on their backs or sides to sleep. In 1996, the AAP revised its recommendation, clarifying that placing infants to sleep on their backs provides the greatest protection against SIDS and is the preferred sleep position.

NICHD launched the "Back to Sleep" campaign in 1994 to amplify the message that placing infants on their backs to sleep can reduce the risk of SIDS and save lives.

According to the National SIDS/Infant Death Resource Center, a division of the Health Resources and Services Administration (HRSA) Maternal and Child Health Bureau, the mortality rate from SIDS decreased dramatically (nearly 40%) between 1995 and 2001 (**Table 14-7**).

Table 14-7 SIDS Mortality Rates 1995–2001[1] (All Races)

Rates per 100,000 live births	
1995	87.2
1996	78.5
1997	77.2
1998	71.7
1999	66.8
2000	62.1
2001[1]	55.5

[1] Last year with complete and final data.

In addition to promoting the "Back to Sleep" campaign, prehospital professionals can further reduce the risk of SIDS by educating new parents to routinely practice the following when placing their baby to sleep:

- Make sure that everyone who cares for the baby (ie, babysitters, relatives) puts the baby to sleep on his or her back.
- Use a firm, tight-fitting mattress in a crib that meets current safety standards.
- Remove pillows, quilts, comforters, stuffed toys, and other soft products from the crib.
- Dress the baby in the appropriate sleep clothing so that other covering will be unnecessary.
- Place the baby so that his or her feet are at the bottom of the crib.
- Make sure the baby's head remains uncovered during sleep.
- Keep the baby warm, but not too warm.
- Make sure that everyone who cares for the baby understands the dangers of soft bedding.
- Avoid adult beds, waterbeds, sofas, or other soft surfaces for sleep.

Support of campaigns against cigarette smoking is also important. Recent research has shown that the risk of SIDS doubles among infants exposed to cigarette smoke after birth, and triples for infants exposed both during pregnancy and after birth. Because formula feeding is a possible risk factor for SIDS, new mothers should be encouraged to breastfeed, if possible.

6. What are some healthy practices for the EMS provider following the sudden death of a child?

There is no doubt that the sudden, unexpected death of a child is an emotionally traumatic event for even the most experienced EMS provider. Although experienced in dealing with the death of an adult resulting from illness, accidents, or even homicide, you may be surprised at the depth of your feelings regarding a child's death.

Responses of the EMS provider to the sudden and unexpected death of a child may include one or more of the following:

- Anger or blame
- Personal identification with the parents or caregivers
- Withdrawal
- Avoidance of the parents or caregiver
- Self-doubt
  - If resuscitation is attempted and the baby is unable to be resuscitated
- Sadness and depression

There are many ways to decrease the impact of stress associated with the death of an infant or child. Critical incident stress debriefing (CISD) or other support groups may help EMS personnel cope with the death of a child. CISD sessions often are conducted within 24 to 72 hours following an incident.

Other techniques that may help decrease the stress response to the sudden death of a child include the following:

- Talk to your supervisor or coworkers and share your feelings.
- Exercise, plan leisure time, and limit overtime hours; maintain a balanced lifestyle outside of work.
- Seek support from SIDS or infant death specialists at the local or state health department.
- Further your education about SIDS.
  - For more information regarding SIDS, contact the following agencies:
    - National SIDS Alliance: 1-800-221-SIDS
    - American SIDS Institute: *www.sids.org*
- Get adequate rest and eat a balanced diet.
- Avoid the use of drugs or alcohol.
- Seek religious or peer counseling.
- Request personal psychological assistance.

It is important for the EMS provider to realize that SIDS babies cannot be resuscitated because most infants are not discovered until well after they have died. Although clearly a tragic event, babies who die from SIDS do so in their sleep with no signs of suffering.

Summary

Sudden infant death syndrome (SIDS) is the sudden and unexpected death of an infant under one year of age that remains unexplained after a thorough postmortem evaluation, including performance of a complete autopsy, examination of the death scene, and review of the clinical history. Although the number of SIDS deaths has declined over the past 10 years, it remains the leading cause of death in infants between 1 month and 1 year of age. SIDS is rare within the first month of life.

SIDS cannot be predicted or prevented; however, a number of risk factors have been identified. As a prehospital professional, you should educate the public regarding ways to reduce the risk of SIDS. The reduction in the number of SIDS cases is most likely attributed to the "Back to Sleep" campaign, which is based on the American Academy of Pediatrics' recommendation to place infants on their backs when they sleep.

In most cases, the infant with SIDS has been dead for an extended period of time and resuscitative efforts are not indicated. You must project an empathetic, professional, and nonjudgmental demeanor when communicating the infant's death to the parents or caregivers. Express your condolences and determine if the parents wish to have additional support at the scene (eg, relatives, clergy). Additionally, you must be aware of your own feelings and seek support or counseling as needed. The death of a child can be a source of significant stress for the prehospital professional, regardless of his or her years of experience in EMS.

Because SIDS can only be diagnosed by a medical examiner through the performance of an autopsy, the information you obtain and factually document regarding the infant's death and observations made at the scene will be valuable in determining the cause of death.

15

9-Year-Old Male Near-Drowning Victim

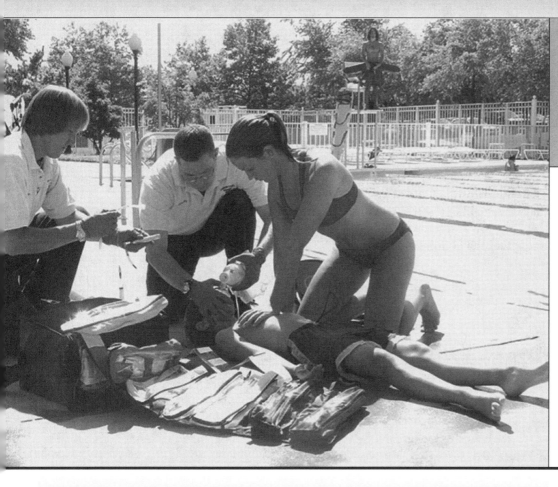

At 3:10 PM, you receive a call for "CPR in progress" at the city park's swimming pool. You and your partner immediately respond to the scene, approximately 5 minutes from your station. A second paramedic ambulance is simultaneously dispatched to the scene.

Upon arrival, you find a lifeguard performing one-rescuer CPR on the patient, a 9-year-old male. The lifeguard states that she did not witness the child's submersion, but says that he couldn't have been under the water for more than 5 minutes. You ask the lifeguard to stop CPR as you perform an initial assessment (**Table 15-1**). Your partner manually stabilizes the child's head in a neutral in-line position.

Table 15-1 Initial Assessment

Level of Consciousness	Unconscious and unresponsive
Mechanism of Injury	Submersion injury; unwitnessed mechanism
Airway and Breathing	Airway is patent; respirations, absent
Circulation	Carotid pulse, absent; skin, cool and pale; no gross bleeding

1. On the basis of the information obtained thus far, what are your treatment priorities?

_____

_____

_____

_____

The child is displaying the cardiac rhythm shown in **Figure 15-1**. Reassessment reveals that he remains pulseless and apneic. The second paramedic unit arrives and begins assisting you and your partner in the management of the child. You ask the lifeguard to contact the child's parents.

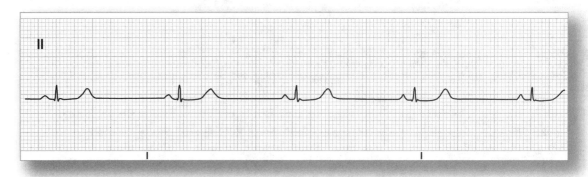

■ **Figure 15-1** Your patient's cardiac rhythm.

2. How will you proceed with the management of this child?

_____

_____

_____

_____

Your partner and a paramedic assistant have appropriately secured the child's airway. As CPR is continuing, you consider your next treatment modality. The lifeguard advises you that the child's mother is en route to the scene. You glance at the cardiac monitor, which remains unchanged.

3. What drugs and dosages are indicated for this child's condition?

_____

_____

_____

_____

4. What are some potentially reversible causes of this child's condition?

_____

_____

_____

With resuscitative efforts ongoing, full spinal motion restriction precautions are taken and the child is quickly loaded into the ambulance. His mother arrives at the scene shortly before your departure and is secured in the front seat of the ambulance by your partner.

5. On the basis of this child's particular situation, what are the most likely causes of his condition? How will you treat them or rule them out?

_____

_____

_____

You continue aggressive resuscitative efforts en route to the hospital, approximately 10 minutes away. Your partner directs your attention to the child's cardiac rhythm, which has changed (**Figure 15-2**). The child now has a weak carotid pulse that corresponds with the rate on the cardiac monitor. Reassessment of the child's airway and breathing reveals that he remains apneic, so ventilatory support is continued. His blood pressure is 60/40 mm Hg.

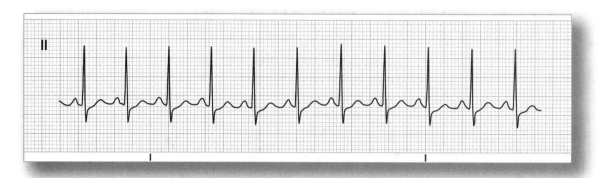

■ **Figure 15-2** Your patient's cardiac rhythm has changed.

6. What further management is indicated for this child?

_____

_____

_____

_____

Following the appropriate post-resuscitation care, the child's condition continues to improve. With an estimated time of arrival at the hospital of 4 minutes, you perform an ongoing assessment (**Table 15-2**) and then call your radio report to the receiving facility.

Table 15-2 Ongoing Assessment

Level of Consciousness	Occasional eye movement is noted; the child is spontaneously moving all four extremities.
Airway and Breathing	Occasional spontaneous breaths are noted; ventilatory support is continued.
Blood Pressure	88/60 mm Hg (with inotropic support)
Pulse	130 beats/min; strong and regular at the carotid artery
Oxygen Saturation	98% (with ventilatory support and 100% oxygen)
Blood Glucose	105 mg/dL
Pupils	Dilated and slow to react
ECG	Sinus tachycardia at 130 beats/min

The child is delivered to the emergency department in stable condition. He is immediately evaluated by the ED physician and a staff pediatrician. Following additional stabilization in the ED, the child is admitted to the pediatric ICU, where he later recovered.

CASE STUDY ANSWERS AND SUMMARY

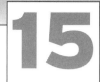

1. On the basis of the information obtained thus far, what are your treatment priorities?

■ **Maintain manual stabilization of the child's head.**
- Because this child's submersion was not witnessed, the possibility of a spinal injury cannot be ruled out. Therefore, you must direct your partner to maintain manual in-line stabilization of the child's head until full spinal motion restriction precautions (eg, cervical collar, spine board, lateral cervical spine immobilization device) have been taken.

Although the child's airway is clear of water or other secretions at the present time, you must be prepared for the passive regurgitation of copious amounts of water. Have your suction unit immediately available!

■ **Dry the child off and assess his cardiac rhythm.**
- Because the child is pulseless and apneic, assessing the need for defibrillation has priority over CPR—just as it would if the patient were an adult. To assess the child's cardiac rhythm, you must first dry his chest off. Then, you can apply the ECG leads, use the "quick-look" technique with the defibrillation paddles, or apply defibrillation pads.
  - Although ventricular fibrillation (V-fib) and pulseless ventricular tachycardia (V-tach) are less common in children than adults, any patient in cardiac arrest, regardless of his or her age, must be assessed to determine if defibrillation is indicated. If either of these lethal ventricular arrhythmias is observed, defibrillation—an intervention that is just as critical in children with V-fib or pulseless V-tach as it is in adults—must be performed without delay.

2. How will you proceed with the management of this child?

The child's cardiac rhythm displays a sinus bradycardia at approximately 45 beats/min; however, because he is pulseless, his condition is known as pulseless electrical activity (PEA). In addition to continuing CPR, further management should consist of:

■ **Endotracheal intubation**
- After adequate preoxygenation with a bag-valve-mask device and 100% oxygen, the child's airway must be secured with an endotracheal tube as soon as possible. Intubation will definitively protect the child's airway from aspiration, allow for the delivery of 100% oxygen directly into the lungs, and can serve as a route for the administration of certain medications if vascular access is not available.
  - To minimize the risk of regurgitation, and to facilitate visualization of the vocal cords, have your partner apply posterior pressure to the cricoid cartilage (Sellick maneuver).
- Following successful intubation—including confirming proper placement and securing the ET tube—ventilate the pulseless and apneic child at a rate of 8 to 10 breaths/min. At this point, CPR should be performed asynchronously (no pause in compressions to deliver ventilations).
  - Avoid excessive ventilation rates during CPR, whether the child is intubated or not. Excessive ventilation is detrimental because it impedes venous return, thus decreasing cardiac output, cerebral blood flow, and coronary perfusion by increasing intrathoracic pressure.

Aggressive airway management for this child cannot be overemphasized. During the panic phase that occurs prior to submersion, patients commonly swallow large amounts of water. This, and the gastric distention that occurs during basic positive-pressure ventilations (eg, bag-valve-mask, mouth-to-mask), significantly increases the risk of passive regurgitation and aspiration.

Even after the child has been successfully intubated, you should consider inserting a nasogastric (NG) tube and suctioning gastric contents if allowed by locally established protocols (**Figure 15-3**). Significant amounts of water or air in the stomach may force the diaphragm upward and decrease your ability to deliver adequate tidal volume. This can be particularly problematic in infants and children.

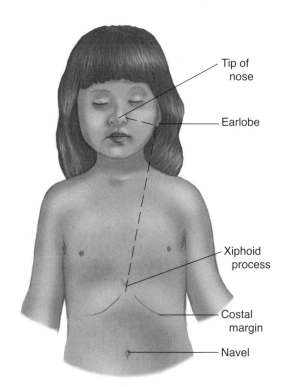

Tip of
nose

Earlobe

Xiphoid
process

Costal
margin

Navel

■ **Figure 15-3** Technique for measuring the distance to insert an NG tube.

Thermal management is also an important consideration for this child. You must ensure that his wet clothes are removed, he is thoroughly dried off, and he is covered with a blanket. Because hypothermia decreases the metabolic rate, cardiac medications will take longer to reach the central circulation and exert their effect. This will decrease the overall effectiveness of your resuscitative efforts. Remember that children are more prone to hypothermia than adults.

■ **Vascular access**
  • Insert an 18- or 20-gauge IV catheter into the most readily accessible vein, usually the antecubital vein.
  • If IV access cannot be obtained within 3 attempts *or* 90 seconds, insert an intraosseous catheter in the child's proximal tibia.

3. What drugs and dosages are indicated for this child's condition?
After a medication route has been obtained, the first drug indicated for PEA is epinephrine. The dosing regimen depends on the route by which the drug is administered:

■ **Intravenous or intraosseous**
  • 0.01 mg/kg (0.1 mL/kg) of a 1:10,000 solution

■ **Endotracheally**
  • 0.1 mg/kg (0.1 mL/kg) of a 1:1,000 solution

Regardless of the route administered, epinephrine should be circulated with effective CPR and repeated every 3 to 5 minutes as needed. Higher doses of epinephrine may be indicated in certain situations. Contact medical control or follow locally established protocols as needed.

4. What are some potentially reversible causes of this child's condition?

Pulseless electrical activity (PEA) is not a specific cardiac rhythm; it is a condition in which any cardiac rhythm (except for V-fib or pulseless V-tach) appears on the cardiac monitor, but does not produce a palpable pulse. Although effective CPR, airway management, and drug therapy are essential treatments for any patient in cardiac arrest, the critical point is that PEA may be reversible if an underlying cause is *quickly identified and promptly treated*. **Table 15-3** lists the potentially reversible causes of PEA. Without rapid identification and treatment of the underlying cause(s) of PEA, the rhythm will deteriorate to asystole and the child will die.

Table 15-3 Potentially Reversible Causes of PEA[1]

Hypovolemia
Hypoxia
Hydrogen ions (acidosis)
Hyper-/hypokalemia
Hypoglycemia
Hypothermia
Toxins (eg, poisons, drugs)
Tamponade (cardiac)
Tension pneumothorax
Thrombosis (coronary and pulmonary)
Trauma

[1] *The above-listed conditions are not all inclusive of the potential underlying causes of PEA; a careful assessment is therefore critical.*

5. On the basis of this child's particular situation, what are the most likely causes of his condition? How will you treat them or rule them out?

Because the child was submerged in water, it is likely that his condition is the combined result of hypoxia, hypothermia, and acidosis—especially since the rate of his cardiac rhythm is slow. However, without knowing his medical history and the events that preceded the submersion, a careful assessment and maintenance of a high index of suspicion are essential. For example, it would not be unreasonable to administer a 20-mL/kg bolus of an isotonic crystalloid solution—after auscultating breath sounds—to rule out hypovolemia.

In addition to continuing CPR, airway management, and epinephrine every 3 to 5 minutes, further treatment for this child should focus on the following conditions:

■ Hypoxia
  • Is the ET tube still correctly placed?
    ○ Reauscultate breath sounds and the epigastrium.
    ○ Use a secondary confirmation device (eg, capnometry or capnography, esophageal bulb device).
    ○ Note the centimeter marking on the ET tube at the child's teeth.
  • Are there secretions in the ET tube? Is tracheal suctioning indicated?
  • Is the rate of ventilation appropriate for the child's age?
    ○ 8–10 breath/min in the pulseless and apneic child
  • Is the oxygen flowmeter set at 15 L/min? Is there oxygen in the tank?

■ Acidosis
  • Ensure effective oxygenation and ventilation *first!*
  • Consider sodium bicarbonate (1 to 2 mEq/kg) via IV or IO administration.
    ○ Contact medical control or follow local protocol regarding sodium bicarbonate administration.

- Hypothermia
  - Assess core body temperature (if possible).
  - Remove wet clothing and cover with a blanket (passive external rewarming).
    - Some protocols advocate placement of chemical heat packs at the groin and axillae. Follow local protocols or contact medical control as needed.
  - Warm the patient compartment of the ambulance.

Although certain aspects of cardiac arrest management are standard (eg, CPR, intubation, epinephrine), the treatment of PEA *must* focus on identifying and correcting any potentially underlying causes. If you do not look, you will not find; if you do not find, you cannot treat!

Rapidly transport the child to the closest appropriate facility. Early hospital notification is an essential element as this will allow receiving personnel to adequately prepare for the child's arrival.

6. What further management is indicated for this child?

The key to successful post-resuscitation management is to perform *frequent* cardiopulmonary assessments, with emphasis on the following postarrest treatment interventions:

- **Assess and continue to support oxygenation and ventilation.**
  - Attach a pulse oximeter and monitor the child's SaO$_2$.
    - Remember that adequate peripheral perfusion is necessary to obtain a reliable SaO$_2$ reading. Consider attaching the pulse oximeter probe to the child's earlobe.
- **Assess and maintain adequate perfusion.**
  - 20-mL/kg crystalloid fluid boluses (up to 3)
  - Dopamine (2 to 20 μg/kg/min) via IV/IO infusion if crystalloid boluses are unsuccessful
    - Start at 5 to 10 μg/kg/min for hypotension.
    - Other inotropic or vasoactive drugs may be indicated based on locally established protocols or a direct order from medical control.
- **Continue to maintain body temperature.**
  - Reassess the child's core body temperature if possible.
  - Continue passive external rewarming.
- **Assess blood glucose levels and treat with IV dextrose as needed.**
  - Treat blood glucose levels of less than 60 mg/dL with 1 to 2 mL/kg of 50% dextrose in water (D$_{50}$W).
    - Reassess the blood glucose to: (1) ensure that it has increased to a normal level, and (2) ensure that you have not inadvertently induced hyperglycemia; this may negatively impact the child's neurologic outcome.

During transport, you must continue to perform *frequent* cardiopulmonary assessments. Be alert for conditions that can cause acute deterioration of the child's condition, such as ET tube displacement, ET tube obstruction, pneumothorax, and equipment failure. It is ideal to maintain two functional IV lines—one for fluid resuscitation and the other to administer a continuous medication infusion, if needed.

If time permits, you should perform a detailed physical examination on the child to detect conditions that may have caused or contributed to his condition.

It is optimum to transport the child to a facility that specializes in pediatric critical care; however, if such a facility is not within a reasonable distance, the child should be transported to the closest appropriate facility where he or she can be further stabilized and then transferred to a tertiary facility. If the closest appropriate facility is a considerable distance from the scene, consider requesting air-medical transport.

Summary

Cardiopulmonary arrest in infants and children is rarely a primary event; it is typically associated with factors such as electrocution, trauma, or water-related incidents. This case study depicted a child who was submerged in water for approximately 5 minutes and experienced cardiopulmonary arrest, most likely secondary to the combined effects of hypoxia, hypothermia, and acidosis.

Immediate treatment for a submersion victim is to ensure your own safety and then remove the patient from the water. Protect the patient's cervical spine if trauma is suspected or cannot be ruled out; this can be performed while the patient is still in the water. Once the patient has been removed from the water, perform an initial assessment and treat immediate threats to airway, breathing, or circulation. If the patient is pulseless and apneic, immediate evaluation of his or her cardiac rhythm is crucial in order to identify and treat lethal ventricular arrhythmias.

Treatment for PEA in pediatric patients includes CPR, aggressive airway management, epinephrine every 3 to 5 minutes, and a careful assessment to identify and treat the underlying cause(s) of the PEA. Hypothermia is a potentially reversible cause of PEA; therefore, it is critical to prevent further heat loss and to keep the child warm. Treat hypoxia and acidosis by ensuring airway patency and adequate oxygenation and ventilation *first*; sodium bicarbonate may be indicated per local protocol or direct medical control. Submersion victims commonly swallow large amounts of water during the panic phase; therefore, suction must be readily available if passive regurgitation occurs, especially before the child can be intubated.

Post-resuscitation care involves performing frequent assessments of the child's cardiopulmonary status and maintaining adequate oxygenation, ventilation, and perfusion. Carefully monitor the child's hemodynamic status, be prepared for acute deterioration, and promptly transport him or her to the closest appropriate facility.

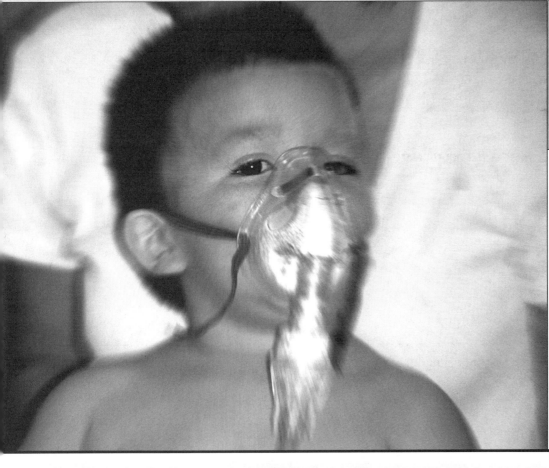

CASE STUDY

16

6-Year-Old Male with an Altered Mental Status

At 5:40 PM, your unit is dispatched to 411 East Third Street for a 6-year-old male with an altered mental status. You and your partner respond to the scene, with a response time of approximately 6 minutes. En route, the dispatcher advises you that the child is conscious and breathing.

1. What are some potential causes of altered mental status in a child?

_____

_____

_____

You arrive at the scene at 5:46 PM. As you enter the residence, you see the child sitting on the couch. He is conscious, but clearly appears ill. His respirations are rapid and appear deep. You perform an initial assessment (**Table 16-1**) as your partner opens the jump kit and prepares to begin treatment.

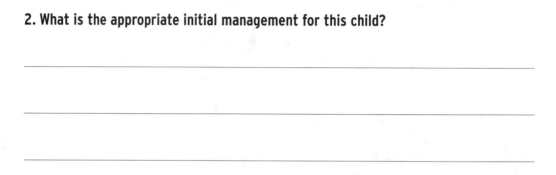

Table 16-1 Initial Assessment

Level of Consciousness	Conscious, but appears confused; not fearful of your presence
Chief Complaint	According to the mother, "He has been ill for the past few days. I thought that it was the flu at first, but then noticed that he was not acting right. That's when I called 9-1-1."
Airway and Breathing	Airway is patent; respirations are rapid and deep.
Circulation	Radial pulses, rapid and weak; skin, warm and dry with poor turgor; no gross bleeding

2. What is the appropriate initial management for this child?

_____

_____

_____

_____

As your partner is performing the appropriate initial treatment for the child, he notes a sweet, fruity odor on the child's breath. A blood glucose reading is obtained; the glucometer reads "high." You ask the mother if her son has diabetes, but she denies this. With information provided by the child's mother, you perform a focused history and physical examination (**Table 16-2**).

Table 16-2 Focused History and Physical Examination

Onset	"He became ill about two days ago and has gotten worse since then."
Duration	"This started about two days ago."
Associated Symptoms	He has been drinking a lot of water, but goes to the bathroom a lot. He also looks like he has lost some weight. Last night, he was complaining that his stomach hurt."
Evidence of Trauma	No gross signs of trauma; mother denies a history of trauma
Interventions Prior to EMS Arrival	None
Seizures	None
Fever	Axillary temperature, 99.4°F
Blood Glucose	The glucometer reads "high."

3. What is the pathophysiology of this child's suspected condition?

_____

_____

_____

_____

The child remains conscious and is tolerating the oxygen mask. As your partner retrieves the stretcher from the ambulance, you obtain baseline vital signs and a SAMPLE history (**Table 16-3**). The mother provides you with her son's medical history.

Table 16-3 Baseline Vital Signs and SAMPLE History

Blood Pressure	88/56 mm Hg
Pulse	130 beats/min, weak and regular
Respirations	40 breaths/min and deep
Oxygen Saturation	97% (on 100% oxygen)
Signs and Symptoms	Abnormal mentation, tachypnea, polyuria, polydipsia, hyperglycemia
Allergies	Penicillin
Medications	None
Pertinent Past History	None
Last Oral Intake	"I gave him some water about 30 minutes ago. The last meal that he ate was about 12 hours ago."
Events Leading to Present Illness	Onset of excessive thirst and urination, progressing to abnormal mentation

4. What specific prehospital care is indicated for this child's condition?

_____

_____

_____

_____

After establishing an IV of normal saline and administering the appropriate fluid volume, you begin transport to a hospital located 15 miles away. En route, the child remains conscious but confused. He converses with you, but is slow to respond to your questions. After performing an ongoing assessment (**Table 16-4**), you call in your radio report to the receiving facility.

Table 16-4 Ongoing Assessment

Level of Consciousness	Conscious, confused, slow to answer questions
Airway and Breathing	Airway remains patent; respirations, 36 breaths/min and deep
Oxygen Saturation	98% (on 100% oxygen)
Blood Pressure	84/52 mm Hg
Pulse	130 beats/min and regular, appears to be stronger
Blood Glucose	Glucometer reads "high."
ECG	Sinus tachycardia at 130 beats/min

The child is delivered to the emergency department and you give a verbal report to the attending physician. Further assessment is performed by the physician, including a serum glucose level, which reads 450 mg/dL. The child is admitted to the pediatric ICU and is provided the appropriate treatment for his condition.

5. What treatment will likely be performed in the emergency department?

_____

_____

_____

_____

16

1. What are some potential causes of altered mental status in a child?

As with the adult, the underlying causes of an altered mental status in children are numerous. In the child, mental status alterations can range from decreased interactiveness or irritability to complete unresponsiveness. Sometimes, the only information that you are provided by the parent or caregiver is that the child is "not acting right." Clearly, such nonspecific information from the caregiver requires a thorough and careful assessment.

Some underlying causes of an altered mental status, such as hypoglycemia, are relatively easy to correct once identified. Other causes, however, may not be so easy to identify because of their obscure or atypical presentation and/or lack of information provided by the parent or caregiver.

When responding to such a call, it is important for the paramedic to recall the common causes of an altered mental status, focusing on some of the most easily correctable ones (eg, hypoglycemia, hypoxia). The AEIOUTIPPS mnemonic is a valuable tool that should routinely be used when attempting to identify the underlying cause(s) of an altered mental status (**Table 16-5**).

Table 16-5 Possible Causes of Altered Mental Status

Alcohol
Epilepsy, endocrine, electrolytes
Insulin (eg, hyper- or hypoglycemia)
Opiates and other drugs
Uremia
Trauma, temperature (eg, fever, environmental exposure)
Infection
Psychogenic
Poison
Shock, stroke, space-occupying intracranial lesion, subarachnoid hemorrhage

It is important to note that, as previously mentioned, some causes of an altered mental status can be successfully treated in the prehospital setting, while others require a more in-depth evaluation (eg, blood analysis, CT scan) and can only be treated in the hospital setting. Therefore, if you have ruled out (or treated) potential causes of the child's condition and little or no clinical improvement is noted, you must prepare for immediate transport to the closest appropriate facility while maintaining and supporting airway, breathing, and circulatory functions en route.

2. What is the appropriate initial management for this child?

Any patient who presents with an altered mental status should be placed on 100% supplemental oxygen without delay. This child, whose respirations are rapid, is breathing with an increased tidal volume; this is manifesting as respirations that are deep. Therefore, initial treatment for this child should consist of the following:

- **100% oxygen via nonrebreathing mask**
  - Closely monitor the adequacy of the child's respiratory effort. If his respirations become shallow (reduced tidal volume), ventilatory assistance with a bag-valve-mask device and 100% oxygen should be initiated.

Remember that minute volume (the amount of air moved through the lungs each minute) can be affected by tidal volume (volume of air moved into or out of the lungs per breath), respiratory rate, or both. Infants and children are often unable to maintain an increased respiratory rate and depth for extended periods of time before becoming physically exhausted. Therefore, a decrease in the rate and depth of an ill child's respirations should alert the paramedic that his or her condition is deteriorating, not necessarily improving.

3. What is the pathophysiology of this child's suspected condition?

This child's clinical presentation is consistent with new-onset type 1 diabetes mellitus (DM), a metabolic condition in which very little, if any, insulin is produced by the pancreas. Because type 1 DM most commonly occurs at a young age, it is also referred to as juvenile-onset DM. The term insulin-dependent diabetes mellitus (IDDM) is used to describe patients who require daily insulin injections to maintain an adequate balance of intravascular and intracellular glucose, but the nomenclature "type 1" is preferred over "juvenile onset" and "insulin-dependent."

Many cases of type 1 DM are hereditary; however, the exact cause of the disease is often unclear. Possible etiologic factors include viral infections, the production of antibodies against the pancreatic beta cells (autoimmune disease), or premature deterioration of the pancreatic beta cells. Regardless of the underlying cause, the result is the same—insufficient insulin to promote the cellular uptake of glucose from the bloodstream.

The clinical presentation of patients with new-onset type 1 DM is that of hyperglycemia and diabetic ketoacidosis (DKA). Hyperglycemia is defined as a blood glucose level greater than 120 mg/dL; DKA is characterized by significant hyperglycemia (blood glucose usually > 200 mg/dL), acidosis (pH < 7.35), and the presence of ketones in the blood or urine.

During the early phase of DKA, hyperglycemia occurs due to a lack of insulin; insulin deficiency inhibits the cellular uptake of glucose from the bloodstream. Inadequate or absent cellular glucose results in two physiologic effects: gluconeogenesis and the formation of ketone bodies (**Figure 16-1**). Gluconeogenesis, a compensatory mechanism of the body to provide new glucose to cells, further elevates blood glucose levels. The

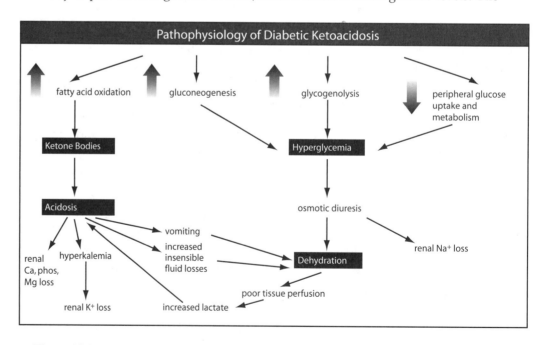

■ **Figure 16-1** Pathophysiology of diabetic ketoacidosis

Figure 16-1: Adapted from Behrman RE, Kliegman RM. *Nelson Essentials of Pediatrics*, 4th Edition. Philadelphia, PA: W.B. Saunders; 2002:185.

Case Study 16: Answers and Summary

formation of ketone bodies is a compensatory mechanism to provide an alternate energy substrate for the brain. Ketone body formation, the result of cellular fat breakdown, can cause ketoacidosis (a type of metabolic acidosis) in the setting of type 1 DM if excess ketone bodies accumulate and cause a drop in the pH of the blood. Therefore, gluconeogenesis and ketone body formation can lead to two negative outcomes in the setting of type 1 DM: hyperglycemia and ketoacidosis.

Excessive blood glucose levels promote an osmotic diuresis in an attempt to rid the body of that excess glucose. With this diuresis comes the loss of large amounts of body water and key electrolytes (eg, sodium, potassium) and subsequent dehydration, sometimes to the point of hypovolemic shock. In severe cases, electrolyte derangements can result in life-threatening cardiac arrhythmias.

The respiratory system attempts to rid the blood of excess ketones by increasing the rate and depth of breathing. This characteristic pattern of tachypnea and hyperpnea, called Kussmaul respirations, is accompanied by a fruity or acetone breath odor; this signifies the excretion of blood acetone via the lungs.

Relative to severe hypoglycemia (insulin shock), the onset of DKA is slow, usually occurring over a period of 12 to 24 hours or longer. Early signs and symptoms include excessive urination (polyuria), excessive hunger (polyphagia), excessive thirst (polydipsia), malaise, and clinical signs of dehydration (eg, tachycardia, poor skin turgor, dry mucous membranes). Later signs of DKA include Kussmaul respirations, an altered mental status, and metabolic acidosis. It is at this point that the patient is said to be in "diabetic coma." The signs and symptoms of DKA are summarized in **Table 16-6**.

Table 16-6 Signs and Symptoms of Diabetic Ketoacidosis

Hyperglycemia (blood glucose usually > 200 mg/dL) • Blood glucose levels in excess of 300 mg/dL are not uncommon.
Polyuria, polydipsia, and polyphagia (The "3 Ps")
Weight loss, nausea, vomiting, and malaise
Abdominal pain
Signs of dehydration • Tachycardia • Poor skin turgor • Warm, dry skin • Dry mucous membranes
Kussmaul respirations
Lethargy

4. What specific prehospital care is indicated for this child's condition?

Prehospital treatment for suspected diabetic ketoacidosis begins by maintaining a patent airway and supporting oxygenation and ventilation. Although Kussmaul respirations often present with deep, rapid breathing, respirations may become shallow and will therefore require some form of positive-pressure ventilation to maintain adequate minute volume. Comatose children should be intubated to achieve definitive airway protection.

For children with signs of mild to moderate dehydration, an infusion of isotonic crystalloid is appropriate; a one-time bolus of 20 mL/kg (IV or IO) is indicated if the child is experiencing signs of hypoperfusion (eg, weak peripheral pulses, delayed capillary refill, hypotension). After that, slow correction of dehydration with IV fluid is important in children due to a higher risk of cerebral edema with aggressive fluid resuscitation. Therefore, administering isotonic fluid such as normal saline or lactated Ringer's solution at a maintenance rate is the best approach in the setting of compensated hypovolemic shock.

Although rarely given in the prehospital setting, medical control may order regular insulin via IV or SC administration in extenuating circumstances (eg, prolonged transport, the patient has prescribed insulin).

Because of the dehydration associated with ketoacidosis, the loss of key electrolytes (eg, potassium, sodium) may result in potentially life-threatening cardiac arrhythmias. Therefore, the child's cardiac rhythm should be monitored.

On occasion, it may be difficult to distinguish between the symptoms of hyperglycemia and hypoglycemia, especially if a blood glucose level cannot be quickly determined. However, hypoglycemia can be accurately and quickly diagnosed with a bedside glucometer. Glucometer readings in the setting of excessive hyperglycemia may not be accurate. If true hypoglycemia is present, however, 1 to 2 mL/kg of 50% dextrose (D_{50}) should be administered via IV or IO bolus. If the patient is hypoglycemic, glucose is truly what he or she needs and may prevent death.

Rapidly transport the child to an appropriate medical facility where definitive care can be provided. Closely monitor the child's condition en route and contact medical control as needed.

5. What treatment will likely be performed in the emergency department?

Treatment in the emergency department will focus on continued fluid rehydration, lowering circulating blood glucose levels, and treating acidosis and electrolyte abnormalities.

Insulin will be administered via continuous infusion at a rate of 0.05 to 0.1 units/kg/hr. When blood glucose levels fall below 300 mg/dL during treatment, glucose should be added to the IV fluids to prevent hypoglycemia. The insulin infusion rate is usually not decreased until the severity of acidosis has diminished (serum bicarbonate concentration > 15 mEq/L).

The acidosis associated with DKA is caused by ketone production secondary to insulin deficiency and the accumulation of lactate due to dehydration. Treatment with insulin inhibits further ketone production and facilitates the clearance of ketones from the body. IV fluids will correct the dehydration. Therefore, the combination of insulin and IV crystalloids is usually sufficient in the correction of acidosis. The administration of sodium bicarbonate to treat acidosis is controversial at present.

Summary

Diabetic ketoacidosis (DKA) is a potentially life-threatening complication of diabetes mellitus. It is characterized by hyperglycemia and ketone production (with resultant acidosis) secondary to fat-based metabolism. DKA is usually present in patients with new-onset type 1 DM; it can also occur in patients with an established history of type 1 DM (ie, when the patient forgets to take his or her prescribed insulin or inadvertently underdoses).

Early signs of DKA include excessive urination and thirst secondary to the osmotic diuresis caused by elevated serum glucose levels. As DKA progresses, the patient becomes ketoacidodic and develops Kussmaul respirations in an attempt to rid the body of excess blood acetone. Blood glucose levels in excess of 300 mg/dL are not uncommon in patients with DKA.

Prehospital care for the patient with DKA should focus on maintaining airway patency and supporting oxygenation and ventilation. IV or IO access should be obtained and crystalloid fluids given as needed to counteract dehydration. A 20-mL/kg bolus and maintenance IV fluid with isotonic normal saline or lactated Ringer's solution is often needed to treat the child with DKA.

Because definitive therapy (eg, insulin, correction of electrolytes) cannot be provided in the prehospital setting, rapid transport to an appropriate medical facility is essential. Continuously monitor the child en route and observe for cardiac arrhythmias caused by electrolyte derangements.

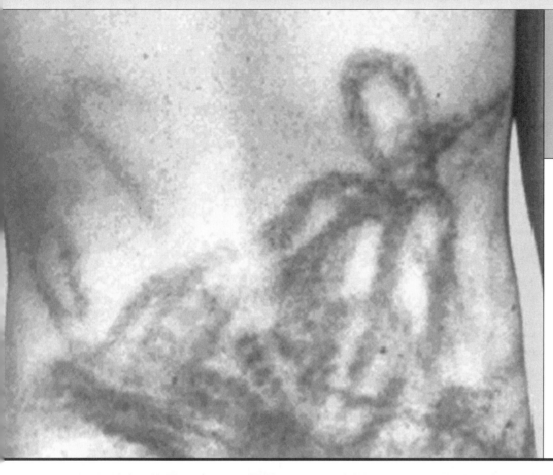

17

A 10-Year-Old Abused Male

At 9:45 PM, you are dispatched to a residence for an "injured child." You and your partner immediately recognize the address as one that you have responded to on several occasions in the past. Because of this, you request that law enforcement respond to the scene. Your response time to the scene is less than 3 minutes.

You arrive at the scene at 9:48 PM and knock on the door of the residence. A young male greets you at the door and identifies himself as the boyfriend of the child's mother. He points to the living room and says, "He's in there." You approach the child, a 10-year-old male, who is sitting quietly on the couch; he is holding his left arm against his chest. When you ask the child what happened, the boyfriend quickly and somewhat rudely interjects by stating, "He fell off his bike again!"

1. What are some common characteristics and behaviors of an abuser?

_____

_____

_____

_____

With the boyfriend watching intently, you perform an initial assessment of the child (**Table 17-1**). When you ask him where he hurts, he wearily looks up at the boyfriend and states, "My left arm hurts." Again, the boyfriend rudely interjects and says, "I told you, he fell off his bike; that's why I called you!"

Table 17-1 Initial Assessment

Mechanism of Injury	According to the boyfriend, "He fell off his bike."
Level of Consciousness	Conscious and alert, but distant
Chief Complaint	"My arm hurts."
Airway and Breathing	Airway is patent; respirations, normal rate and quality
Circulation	Radial pulses, strong and regular; skin, warm and dry; no gross bleeding

As your partner obtains additional information from the boyfriend, you perform a focused physical examination on the child (**Table 17-2**). The boyfriend is clearly more preoccupied with watching you than he is with answering your partner's questions. A police officer arrives at the scene and obtains information from the boyfriend.

Table 17-2 Focused Physical Examination

Injury Location	Deformity to the left midshaft humerus, contusions to the left forearm
Neurovascular	Radial pulse is present and strong; sensory and motor functions, grossly intact.
Other Injuries	Bruises of various colors to the upper back

2. What information should you obtain during the focused history?

_____

_____

_____

_____

You advise the boyfriend that the child should be transported to the hospital. He tells you that he has some errands to run and will not be able to accompany the child to the hospital. After providing you with the phone number of the child's mother, who is at work, he departs the scene. As you are talking to the mother on the phone, your partner obtains baseline vital signs and a SAMPLE history (**Table 17-3**).

Table 17-3 Baseline Vital Signs and SAMPLE History

Blood Pressure	102/62 mm Hg
Pulse	100 beats/min, strong and regular
Respirations	22 breaths/min, adequate depth
Signs and Symptoms	Deformity to the left humerus, contusions to the left forearm, multiple bruises to the upper back
Allergies	According to the child, "I don't know."
Medications	None
Pertinent Past History	None
Last Meal	According to the child, "I can't remember."
Events Leading to Injury	With hesitation, the child tells you, "I fell off my bike."

You have appropriately splinted the child's arm and have received verbal consent from the mother to transport the child to a hospital located approximately 10 miles away. She states that she will meet you at the emergency department.

3. Is a detailed physical examination indicated for this child? If so, why?

_____

_____

_____

_____

The child remains quiet throughout the duration of the transport; he is still reluctant to answer any of your questions. After performing an ongoing assessment (**Table 17-4**), you call your verbal report to the receiving facility.

Table 17-4 Ongoing Assessment

Level of Consciousness	Conscious and alert, but distant
Airway and Breathing	Airway remains patent; respirations, normal rate and depth
Blood Pressure	100/60 mm Hg
Pulse	110 beats/min, strong and regular
Injury Site	Arm is appropriately splinted; distal pulse, present; sensory and motor functions, grossly intact

4. What are some physical indicators of child maltreatment?

_____

_____

_____

_____

5. What legal obligations do you have regarding this call?

_____

_____

_____

_____

The child is delivered to the emergency department in stable condition. You provide a verbal report to the attending physician and apprise her of your suspicions. After completing the patient care form and leaving a copy with the physician, you return to service.

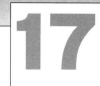

1. What are some common characteristics and behaviors of an abuser?

When assessing a child who has possibly been abused, it is important to assess the caregiver's behavior, both toward the child and toward you. Although child maltreatment occurs in all socioeconomic, religious, and ethnic groups, individuals who abuse children often share some common characteristics and traits.

Common characteristics of people who abuse children include isolation, poor self-concept, a lack of parenting and/or interpersonal skills, and immaturity. They often lack the skills to interact competently with the prehospital care provider. Many times, the abuser was a victim of child abuse.

The characteristics of an abuser often manifest in his or her behavior; therefore, it is important for the provider to note any unusual behavior on the part of the parent or caregiver during his or her assessment of the child. **Table 17-5** lists certain caregiver behaviors that are suggestive of child maltreatment. You should maintain a high index of suspicion if any of these behaviors are observed.

Table 17-5 Caregiver Indicators of Child Maltreatment

Aggressive or defensive attitude when asked about the injury circumstances
Lack of emotion, feeling, or concern regarding the child (apathy)
Overconcern regarding a relatively minor injury; underconcern regarding a more serious injury
The history provided is incompatible with the developmental abilities of the child.
Inconsistent or conflicting account regarding how the injury occurred (if more than one caregiver is present)
An abnormal delay in seeking medical care for the child
Reluctance or refusal to allow you to transport the child
Any bizarre or strange conduct

Some parents or caregivers of injured (non-abused) children may project a demanding or angry demeanor toward EMS personnel who are caring for their child; this is usually a manifestation of fear for the child's well-being. However, the parent or caregiver of a non-abused child often calms down following a simple explanation of what you are doing; this is less likely to occur with the parent or caregiver who has intentionally injured his or her child.

You should be especially concerned when a parent or caregiver refuses to allow you to transport his or her child to the hospital, especially if you have clearly explained the potential seriousness of the injury. Most prudent, caring parents will readily give consent to treatment and transport.

2. What information should you obtain during the focused history?

After stabilizing any immediately life-threatening conditions during the initial assessment, you should obtain a careful history regarding the child's injury or injuries (**Table 17-6**). If maltreatment is suspected, you must exercise caution when questioning the parent or caregiver; do not ask questions in an accusatory manner. However, pay close attention to, and carefully document, the caregiver's comments.

Although the boyfriend in this case study is consistent in his account of how the child was injured, he is the only caregiver present. In cases where more than one caregiver is present, it is important to interview each caregiver, paying particular attention to any inconsistencies regarding the event. Interviewing caregivers separately is more likely to reveal inconsistencies, if any exist. Do not conduct multiple interviews if doing so will unnecessarily delay transport of the child.

Perhaps one of the most significant indicators of an intentionally inflicted injury is when the description of the injury is inconsistent with the circumstances and/or if the injury mechanism is incompatible with the developmental age of the child. For example, it is common for a 10-year-old child to fall from his or her bike; it is not common for a 10-month-old infant to pull a pot of boiling water off of the stove. In this particular case, the injury circumstance seems plausible; however, the behavior of both the child and boyfriend is not consistent with what would typically be expected following an accidental injury.

Table 17-6 Focused History Considerations

How did the injury occur?
- Does the caregiver offer an adequate explanation for the injury?
- Does the history of the injury differ between caregivers or from caregiver to child?
  - Remember, abused children often remain silent for fear of retribution; they tend to "go along" with the caregiver's story.

How long ago did the injury occur?
- Was there an unusually long delay before EMS was notified? If so, what was the reason for the delay?
- Is the appearance of the injury or injuries consistent with the time frame given?

Did anybody witness the injury?
- Was the child being supervised? If so, by whom?
- Are the caregivers and witnesses stories consistent?
  - Accurate information can only be obtained from those who actually witnessed the injury.

Was the child moved to another location after the injury?
- If so, determine why the caregiver felt it was necessary to move the child.

Has the child been injured before?
- You should be especially concerned since you and your partner have responded to this residence several times in the past.
- If possible, recall the nature of the previous calls. Was the same child involved in the previous incident(s)? Is this the same caregiver that was present last time?

Your focused history should also include observations made at the scene, such as the general condition of the residence, the location of the child upon your arrival, and any unsafe or unsanitary conditions.

Careful, objective documentation is absolutely critical when dealing with a case of suspected child maltreatment. Factually document all findings, including your physical assessment of the child, conditions at the scene, and comments made by the child and caregiver. Use quotation marks when documenting statements made by the child and caregiver. Document any treatment provided prior to your arrival.

3. Is a detailed physical examination indicated for this child? If so, why?

Usually, a detailed physical examination is performed on trauma patients with a significant mechanism of injury and on unresponsive medical patients. However, when caring for a child suspected of being abused, a detailed physical examination may reveal other findings and injury patterns that are consistent with an intentionally inflicted injury and should therefore be performed whenever possible. A detailed exam may also reveal signs of chronic maltreatment (eg, old scars, improperly healed fractures). If the child's condition is clinically unstable, however, your focus should remain on the ABCs; in such cases, a detailed exam would have a low priority and would clearly be impractical.

When exposing the child to perform a detailed physical examination, do so in a manner that does not frighten or embarrass him or her. If the caregiver questions why you are examining areas of the child's body not directly affected by the injury, explain that a detailed exam is necessary in order to identify and properly care for all injuries. As previously mentioned, do not make comments or ask questions that may be construed as being accusatory.

Carefully examine all parts of the child's body, noting the presence of bruises, deformities, lacerations, or other signs of injury. If suspicious injuries are discovered, ask the child how he or she acquired them. Recall, however, that many children will not be forthcoming with the truth, especially if the abuser is present.

If possible, conduct your examination in private, away from the parent or caregiver. This can be accomplished as your partner obtains general information about the child from the parent or caregiver in another room. Reassure the child that you are there to help him or her and that he or she can be honest with you regarding what happened.

Because you should remove the child from the abusive environment as soon as possible, the detailed physical exam, if performed, should be accomplished en route to the hospital. Thoroughly document your physical exam findings and any comments made by the child and caregiver.

4. What are some physical indicators of child maltreatment?

As previously discussed, a careful examination of a child who is suspected of being abused is a crucial part of your overall care of the child; it may reveal suggestive injury patterns.

Clearly, you should not respond to every call involving an ill or injured child with the preconceived notion that signs of abuse will be discovered; most of the time the child was indeed injured unintentionally. However, uncharacteristic behavior of the child and caregiver should heighten your index of suspicion and should prompt you to perform a more in-depth physical examination.

When assessing the child, it is important to recall various parts of the child's anatomy where accidental injuries commonly occur. For example, bruises to the shins and knees, especially in toddlers, are relatively common. They often bump into coffee tables and other furniture that is low to the ground. Lacerations to the chin are also common injuries in children. However, these same injuries in infants, who are not yet mobile, may suggest an inflicted injury.

A key physical indicator of abuse is the presence of bruising in inappropriate anatomic areas. Bruises to the back, thighs, buttocks, face, or posterior leg are more likely to be inflicted injuries. Note the color of the bruises; this will give you an estimate of the injury's age (**Table 17-7**).

Table 17-7 Bruises in Various Stages of Healing

Red Indeterminate	
Yellow Older than 18 hours	
Blue, Purple, or Black From 1 hour to resolution	

Source: Langlois NEI, Gresham, GA. The aging of bruises: A review and study of the color changes with time. *Forensic Science International*. 1991; 50:227-228. Reprinted with permission.

When examining bruises of various colors, it is important to remember that injuries inflicted at the same time, on the same child, in the same manner, may appear differently and can heal at a different rate. The size and color of the bruise also depends on the severity of the inflicted injury. As previously discussed, bruises located in areas where children are uncommonly injured are suggestive of inflicted injury (**Figure 17-1**).

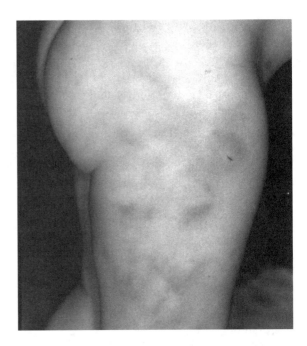

■ **Figure 17-1** Bruises in various stages of healing in inappropriate anatomic areas are suggestive of an inflicted injury.

When examining a child who has experienced burns, pay close attention to the mechanism of injury provided by the caregiver as well as the burn injury itself. For example, a child who pulls a pot of boiling water from the stove is likely to have irregular burns caused by a characteristic splash pattern. Conversely, "stocking/glove" burn patterns indicate that his or her hands or feet were intentionally held in hot water (**Figure 17-2**). Donut burns occur when a child's buttocks are intentionally held in hot water (**Figure 17-3**). With these burn patterns, the child's extremities are usually restrained by the abuser, preventing him or her from thrashing about and splashing; therefore, splash burns are usually absent.

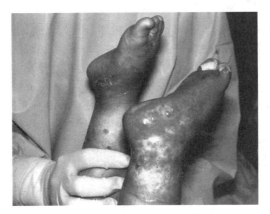

■ **Figure 17-2** Stocking/glove burn patterns of the hands or feet are almost always inflicted injuries.

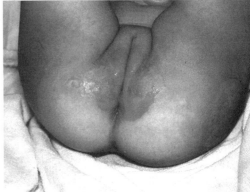

■ **Figure 17-3** A donut burn occurs when a child's buttocks are intentionally held in hot water.

Remember, the mere presence of bruises on a child's body does not necessarily indicate abuse. As a child gets older, his or her ability to do things that might result in injury increases. However, when bruises are found in anatomically unlikely areas, and the mechanism described is inconsistent with the injury pattern, you should become suspicious.

5. What legal obligations do you have regarding this call?

It must be reiterated that the prehospital care provider must never accuse a parent or caregiver of child maltreatment, directly or indirectly. Additionally, questions or comments that suggest such accusations must be avoided. Verbally accusing a parent or caregiver of abusing his or her child may expose the provider to allegations of slander; documenting subjective information or opinionated statements may lead to allegations of libel.

However, in many states, the prehospital care provider is considered a "mandated reporter" and must legally report all suspected cases of child maltreatment to the appropriate authorities. Although some states may not legally require you to report your suspicions, you certainly have a moral obligation.

Under most states laws, the mandated reporter's identity is protected and he or she is afforded protection from liability from false allegations, provided the allegations are made in good faith and are based on reasonable and objective information.

Note that absolute proof of maltreatment is not required, only suspicion. You should report your suspicions to the emergency department physician; some states require EMS personnel to report cases of suspected abuse directly to law enforcement officials.

Whoever your reporting authority is, he or she must report the incident to the local Child Protective Services (CPS) agency, from where the appropriate investigation will be launched. Remember, the intent of reporting suspected cases of child maltreatment is not an attempt to harm or punish a family, but rather an attempt to protect the child.

In some states, there may be legal action brought against the prehospital care provider for not reporting suspected cases of child maltreatment. It is important to be thoroughly familiar with the laws of the state in which you function. It is not within your realm of responsibility to prove that child maltreatment has occurred; however, you must recognize the indicators of abuse, objectively document your physical exam findings and comments made by the child and parent/caregiver, and report your suspicions to the appropriate authorities. It is the responsibility of CPS and, in some cases, law enforcement, to substantiate alleged child maltreatment.

Summary

Child maltreatment is defined as the infliction of intentional harm to a child resulting from inappropriate or abnormal practices. It includes physical, sexual, and emotional abuse, and neglect. In the year 2000, approximately 3 million cases of child maltreatment were reported to the U.S. Department of Health and Human Services; nearly 900,000 of these cases were confirmed. Unfortunately, more than 1,200 deaths were the result of child maltreatment in 2000. Frighteningly, for each case of child maltreatment reported, it is estimated that at least one or two cases are unrecognized or unreported.

Child maltreatment occurs within families of all cultural and socioeconomic backgrounds; it is not limited to low-income families. This case study depicted a child who was physically abused; however, it is important for the prehospital provider to remember that child maltreatment is not limited to outright physical injury.

If you discover indicators of child maltreatment, a thorough examination should be performed. Provide immediate care for all life-threatening injuries and transport the child to an appropriate medical facility as soon as possible.

Pay close attention to the behaviors of the child and caregiver, specifically noting how the child and caregiver interact. Remain alert for suspicious activities, such as inconsistencies in the injury mechanism, injuries that are incompatible with the developmental abilities of the child, suggestive injury patterns, and abnormal delays in calling EMS. Carefully and objectively document your suspicions and report them to the appropriate authorities.

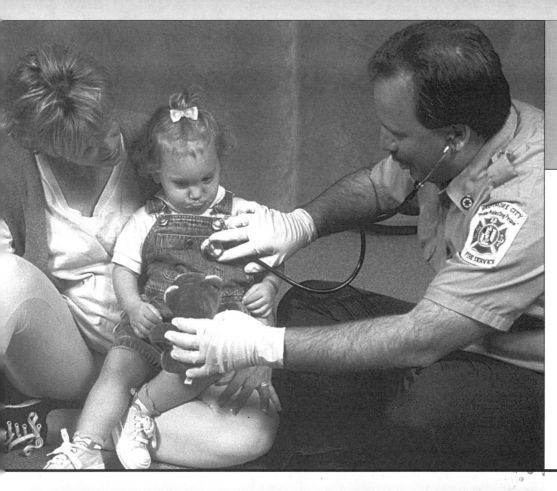

18

2-Year-Old Female with High Fever

At 1:40 AM, you are dispatched to 311 West Kronkosky Street for a child with high fever. You and your partner proceed to the scene with a response time of approximately 5 minutes.

Upon arriving at the scene at 1:45 AM, you are greeted at the door of the residence by a young female holding her child. She tells you that her daughter has been running a fever, but now she is "not acting right." The child, a 2-year-old female, is crying and very irritable. You perform an initial assessment with the child in her mother's arms (**Table 18-1**).

Table 18-1 Initial Assessment

Level of Consciousness	Crying, irritable
Chief Complaint	According to the mother, "Fever and not acting right."
Airway and Breathing	Airway is patent; respirations, increased and unlabored.
Circulation	Radial pulses, rapid and bounding; skin, hot and flushed; capillary refill time, 2 seconds; no gross bleeding

1. What is your initial treatment for this child?

_____

_____

_____

_____

You have completed the appropriate initial treatment for the child. The mother tells you that she is usually easily able to console and calm her daughter by picking her up when she is sick; however, for some reason, the child is not easily consoled this time and actually cries more when she is picked up. You perform a focused history and physical examination (**Table 18-2**) with information provided by the mother.

Table 18-2 Focused History and Physical Examination

Onset	"She started running a fever about a day and a half ago."
Duration	"She has been sick for the last day and a half."
Associated Symptoms	"She has refused to eat anything for the past day or so. Also, I noticed that she has been grabbing the sides of her head; however, she doesn't seem to move her head, she only moves her eyes. She vomited twice in the last 12 hours."
Evidence of Trauma	No gross signs of trauma; mother denies a history of trauma
Seizures	No seizures were observed.
Fever	Rectal temperature, 102.5°F
Interventions Prior to EMS Arrival	"I gave her 1½ tsp of children's ibuprofen about 30 minutes ago."

2. What is your field impression of this child?

_____

_____

_____

_____

3. What are petechiae and purpura? What do they indicate?

_____

_____

_____

_____

The child remains conscious, but is not resistant to your assessment. You advise the mother that the child should be transported to the emergency department; she agrees. Shortly before departing the scene, you obtain a set of baseline vital signs and a SAMPLE history (**Table 18-3**).

Table 18-3 Baseline Vital Signs and SAMPLE History

Blood Pressure	Not obtained
Pulse	120 beats/min, strong and regular
Respirations	36 breaths/min and regular; adequate depth
Oxygen Saturation	98% (on supplemental oxygen)
Signs and Symptoms	Fever, apparent headache and nuchal rigidity, vomiting, irritability
Allergies	None
Medications	None on a regular basis; ibuprofen 30 minutes ago
Pertinent Past History	Recent runny nose and cough
Last Oral Intake	12 hours prior, but promptly vomited
Events Leading to Illness	Recent URI symptoms, followed by onset of fever and irritability

4. What treatment will you provide to this child en route to the hospital?

_____

_____

_____

_____

You secure the child on the stretcher, place mother on the bench seat, and begin transport. En route, you continue oxygen therapy and continuous monitoring of the child. Your transport time is relatively short, so you perform a quick ongoing assessment of the child (**Table 18-4**) and then call your radio report to the receiving facility.

Table 18-4 Ongoing Assessment

Level of Consciousness	Conscious, irritable, crying
Airway and Breathing	Airway remains patent; respirations, 34 breaths/min and unlabored
Oxygen Saturation	98% (on supplemental oxygen)
Blood Pressure	Not obtained
Pulse	124 beats/min, strong and regular

You deliver the child to the emergency department. Upon arrival, you note the development of a fine rash to the child's lower extremities. After giving your verbal report to the attending physician, you complete your patient care form and give a copy to the registration clerk. Subsequent assessment and a lumbar puncture (LP) confirm the condition that you suspected. The child is given antibiotics immediately and is admitted to the hospital.

1. What is your initial treatment for this child?

■ Minimize the child's anxiety

Although the child is clearly ill, your findings in the initial assessment do not warrant immediate separation of her from her mother. If possible, continue your assessment of the child while her mother is holding her. This will minimize the child's anxiety and may facilitate a more accurate assessment.

■ 100% supplemental oxygen
  • Pediatric nonrebreathing mask or blow-by technique

Although the child's respirations are increased, they are unlabored and are producing adequate tidal volume; therefore, ventilatory assistance is not indicated at this point. Administer passive oxygenation in a nonthreatening manner to avoid increasing the child's anxiety. If she becomes more irritable after applying a nonrebreathing mask, have the mother hold oxygen tubing near her nose and mouth.

Continue to monitor the child's respiratory effort and closely observe for signs of inadequate ventilation, such as a shallow depth of breathing (reduced tidal volume) or a decreasing mental status. Be prepared to assist ventilations with a bag-valve-mask device if signs of inadequate breathing are observed.

2. What is your field impression of this child?

This child's clinical presentation is highly suggestive of meningitis. The following signs, symptoms, and historical findings support this field impression:

■ Fever

■ Headache
  • Young children will often grab the sides of their head or place their hand on their head when they are experiencing a headache. Older children are usually able to tell you that their head hurts.

■ Irritability
  • Irritability is a very common sign of meningitis in smaller children. You should be especially suspicious if the child tends to become more irritable when she is picked up (paradoxical irritability); this indicates increased pain as traction is pulled on the inflamed meninges surrounding the spinal cord.

■ Apparent nuchal rigidity (neck stiffness)
  • The fact that the child will not move her head suggests that she is experiencing nuchal rigidity—a classic sign of meningitis.
  • Nuchal rigidity may not be a reliable sign in children less than 18 to 24 months of age.

Meningitis, also referred to as spinal meningitis, is an inflammation of the meningeal layers that surround and protect the brain and spinal cord. The infection can be bacterial, viral, or even fungal in origin. In many cases, meningitis is preceded by upper respiratory infection (URI) symptoms. In the prehospital setting, it is not possible to determine the etiologic pathogen causing the disease (eg, bacterial, viral, fungal); therefore, you should assume the disease to be bacterial in origin (the most life-threatening) until proven otherwise.

Bacterial meningitis remains a significant cause of mortality and morbidity in children. According to the Centers for Disease Control and Prevention (CDC), 3% to 6% of cases of meningitis in children are fatal; 20% of the patients who survive experience hearing loss or other long-term sequelae (eg, neurological impairment).

Relative to viral (aseptic) meningitis, which typically does not pose the risk of permanent neurological damage, bacterial meningitis is a potentially life-threatening infection. It is often associated with an altered mental status, seizures, and increased intracranial pressure (ICP). If left untreated, bacterial meningitis can result in severe sepsis, permanent neurological damage, and even death.

Prior to 1990, *Haemophilus influenzae* type b (Hib) was the most common cause of bacterial meningitis; however, because a vaccine for Hib is now administered to children as part of their routine immunizations, the occurrence of *H. influenzae* has decreased. According to the CDC, the incidence of Hib-related meningitis between 1980 and 1990 was approximately 40 to 100 per 100,000 children under 5 years of age. Since vaccinations against Hib began, the incidence has decreased to 1.3 per 100,000 children in that same age group. *Neisseria meningitidis* (*N. meningitidis*), also called meningococcal meningitis, and *Streptococcus pneumoniae* (also called pneumococcal meningitis) are currently the leading causes of bacterial meningitis in children greater than one month of age. In neonates (birth to 1 month of age), meningitis is usually caused by *Escherichia coli* (*E. coli*), group B streptococcus, or *Listeria monocytogenes*.

Classic signs and symptoms of bacterial meningitis include high fever, headache, and nuchal rigidity (**Figure 18-1**). In infants, the clinical presentation is commonly that of increased irritability, poor feeding, vomiting, a bulging fontanelle (sign of increased ICP), and inconsolability. Because infants and children less than 18 to 24 months of age often lack adequately developed neck musculature, nuchal rigidity may not manifest; therefore, it is an unreliable sign in this age group. Only in children older than 18 to 24 months of age are headache and nuchal rigidity reliable manifestations of meningitis.

The signs and symptoms of meningitis (**Table 18-5**) can develop over several hours or a few days, and may vary depending on the child's age. For example, infants may present with increased irritability, poor feeding, and difficulty in being consoled; older children are often unable to maintain a comfortable position secondary to muscle stiffness.

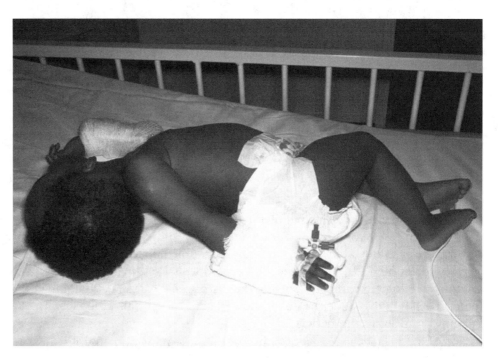

■ **Figure 18-1** Nuchal rigidity is a sign of meningitis, particularly in children older than 18 to 24 months of age.

Case Study 18: Answers and Summary

Table 18-5 Signs and Symptoms of Bacterial Meningitis

Fever
Headache (in children > 18 to 24 months of age)
Nuchal rigidity (in children > 18 to 24 months of age)
Photophobia (sensitivity to light)
Nausea and vomiting • Projectile vomiting may occur with increased ICP.
Irritability/difficult to console • Paradoxical irritability in infants
Bulging fontanelle (in infants)
Decreased level of consciousness/lethargy
Skin rashes • Petechiae or purpura
Seizures

In older children, the inability to extend the legs with the hips flexed (Kernig sign) and/or involuntary flexion of the hip, knee, or ankle when the neck is passively flexed (Brudzinski sign) are suggestive of meningeal irritation. However, the absence of these clinical findings does not rule out meningitis.

Bacterial meningitis is a contagious disease. The primary mode of transmission is via the airborne droplet route, such as the exchange of respiratory secretions (eg, coughing, sneezing, kissing). Unlike the common cold or flu, however, the bacteria are not spread via casual contact with an infected person. Nonetheless, the appropriate BSI precautions—gloves and facial protection—must be strictly followed when caring for a patient with suspected meningitis.

3. What are petechiae and purpura? What do they indicate?

Petechiae are small (< 0.05 cm) circumscribed areas of superficial bleeding into the skin. Initially, they appear as red pinpoint-sized spots and then turn purple or dark blue. A petechial rash (**Figure 18-2**) is not a disease itself, but a manifestation of an underlying problem. The presence of petechiae indicates a low platelet count (thrombocytopenia) and is associated with a severe systemic infection (sepsis).

Approximately 25% of children with meningococcal meningitis develop an erythematous (red) maculopapular rash followed by petechiae or purpura, most commonly located on the extremities. Purpura, also a manifestation of thrombocytopenia, appears as purple circumscribed skin lesions greater than 0.5 cm in size (**Figure 18-3**).

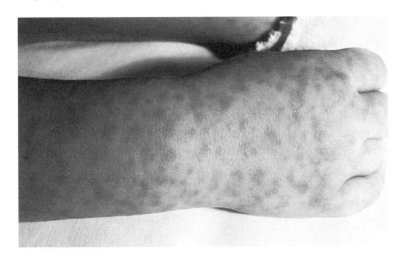

■ **Figure 18-2**
Petechial rash in a child with meningococcal meningitis.

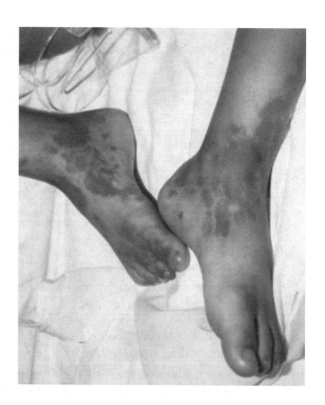

■ Figure 18-3 Purpura in a child with meningococcal meningitis.

Although petechiae and purpura are classically seen in children with meningococcal meningitis, they can also occur in conjunction with other infectious diseases, viral or bacterial.

4. What treatment will you provide to this child en route to the hospital?

Children with suspected meningitis must be closely monitored for the presence of increased intracranial pressure, seizures, and signs of septic shock. Because infants and small children have relatively immature immune systems, they are particularly vulnerable to sepsis.

If respiratory depression develops (suggestive of increased ICP), assist the child's ventilations with a bag-valve-mask device and 100% oxygen. Endotracheal intubation may be necessary if you are unable to provide effective bag-valve-mask ventilations or your transport time to the hospital will be lengthy.

Provided the child remains hemodynamically stable, allow him or her to remain with the caregiver. Continue oxygen therapy as tolerated and promptly transport the child to the hospital. If signs and symptoms of septic shock (**Table 18-6**) are present, obtain IV or IO access and administer 20-mL/kg boluses of normal saline or lactated Ringer's as needed to maintain adequate perfusion. If the child is hemodynamically stable, consider deferring IV therapy until the child is in the emergency department. Remember, you should avoid any unnecessary procedures; these will likely increase the child's anxiety and could cause acute deterioration of his or her clinical condition.

If the child experiences a seizure, administer a benzodiazepine drug such as diazepam (Valium) or midazolam (Versed). If IV or IO access is not available, diazepam can be given via the rectal route; midazolam can be given intramuscularly if needed. Follow locally established protocols or contact medical control as needed regarding the pediatric doses of these drugs.

Table 18-6 Signs and Symptoms of Septic Shock

Weak, rapid peripheral pulses
Rapid, shallow respirations
Poor muscle tone
Cool, pale extremities
• Unless profound peripheral vasoconstriction is present, the child's skin may remain warm or hot secondary to high fever.
Capillary refill time greater than 2 seconds
• Most reliable in children less than 6 years of age
Decreased level of consciousness
• Failure to recognize parents
• Difficult to arouse
Petechial or purpuric rash
Hypotension (late sign)

If, despite two or three crystalloid fluid boluses, the child remains hypotensive, medical control may order an infusion of one of the following vasoactive drugs, both of which should be titrated as necessary to improve perfusion:

- Epinephrine: 0.1 to 1 µg/kg/min
- Dopamine: 2 to 20 µg/kg/min
  - Usual starting dose is 5 to 10 µg/kg/min.

Definitive treatment for a child with meningitis and septic shock involves the administration of antibiotics—an intervention that cannot be provided in the prehospital setting. Therefore, rapid transport to an appropriate medical facility is essential.

Summary

Meningitis remains a significant cause of mortality and morbidity in children. *Neisseria meningitidis* (*N. meningitidis*), or meningococcal meningitis, and *Streptococcus pneumoniae* (also called pneumococcal meningitis), are the most common causes of bacterial meningitis in children older than 1 month of age. *Haemophilus influenzae* type b (Hib) has been virtually eradicated as a cause of bacterial meningitis in children due to Hib vaccinations that began in the late 1980s. If left untreated, bacterial meningitis may result in septic shock, permanent neurological impairment, or death.

Meningitis should be suspected in any child who presents with fever, headache, and nuchal rigidity; however, headache and nuchal rigidity are most reliably assessed in children older than 18 to 24 months of age. Other signs and symptoms include nausea and vomiting, irritability, photophobia, signs of increased intracranial pressure, seizures, and a petechial or purpuric rash. In infants, common signs include paradoxical irritability, poor feeding, a bulging fontanelle, and inconsolability.

Prehospital care for a child with meningitis begins by taking the appropriate BSI precautions, including gloves and facial protection; bacterial meningitis is a contagious disease that is spread by the airborne droplet route. Obtain and maintain the child's airway and provide supplemental oxygen or assisted ventilation as needed. If signs of hypoperfusion are present, 20-mL/kg IV or IO crystalloid fluid boluses should be given. Vasopressor therapy (eg, epinephrine, dopamine) may be required for fluid-refractory hypoperfusion. If the child is hemodynamically stable, consider deferring IV therapy to avoid causing unnecessary anxiety. Promptly transport the child to an appropriate medical facility, while closely monitoring his or her ABCs en route. Meningitis is diagnosed in the emergency department with a lumbar puncture (spinal tap) and is treated definitively with antibiotic therapy.

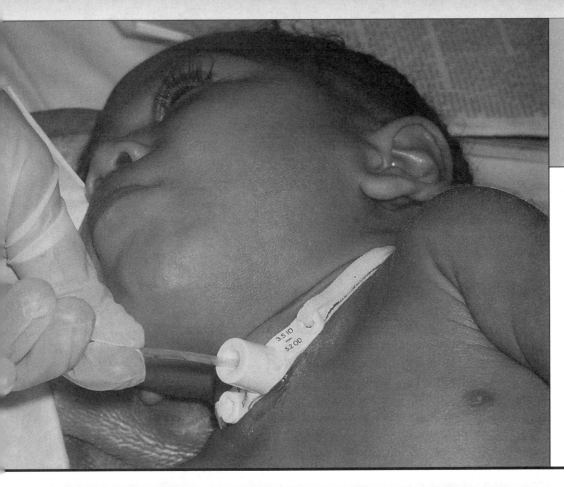

At 2:20 PM, you are dispatched to 518 East Bandera Street for a 3-year-old male with respiratory distress. You have responded several times to this address for the same child, who is on a home ventilator. You and your partner proceed to the scene with a response time of approximately 7 minutes.

You arrive at the scene at 2:27 PM, and are met at the door by the child's mother. As you are being escorted to the child's bedroom, the mother states that her son, who has a tracheostomy tube and is on a home ventilator, suddenly began experiencing respiratory distress about 20 minutes ago. She further states that she suctioned the tracheostomy tube, but this did not seem to correct the problem. As you perform an initial assessment (**Table 19-1**), your partner obtains additional information from the mother.

Table 19-1 Initial Assessment

Level of Consciousness	Intermittently responsive; according to his mother, this is his baseline mental status—he experienced a closed head injury 9 months ago.
Chief Complaint	According to the mother, "He suddenly began working really hard to breathe about 20 minutes ago."
Airway and Breathing	Tracheostomy tube in place; child is on a home ventilator; sternal and intercostal retractions are present.
Circulation	Radial pulses, rapid and regular; skin, cool and dry; no gross bleeding

1. What is a tracheostomy? What are the indications for initial placement of a tracheostomy tube?

_____

_____

_____

As you are assessing the child, the alarm on the mechanical ventilator sounds. The mother tells you that the ventilator was just replaced a week ago. She was trained on the device by the technician; however, the alarm has never sounded before. She becomes panicked and asks you to please do something. The child is still laboring to breathe and his oxygen saturation reads 89%. Your partner attaches a cardiac monitor, which reveals a sinus tachycardia at 130 beats/min.

2. What is your next course of action?

_____

_____

_____

Following your initial attempt to correct the problem, the child's condition has shown little improvement; he is still laboring to breathe. His oxygen saturation is 85% and his heart rate has decreased to 100 beats/min. Your partner, who is ventilating the child, tells you that he is meeting resistance when squeezing the bag. You assess the child's breath sounds; they are equal, but are difficult to hear.

3. What are the most common causes of respiratory distress in children with tracheostomy tubes? How should you proceed with your assessment?

_____

_____

_____

_____

After suctioning the tracheostomy tube, you reassess the child. He is still laboring to breathe and your partner is still meeting resistance during ventilations. The child's breath sounds remain equal but are still difficult to hear. You and your partner agree that the tracheostomy tube should be replaced.

4. What is the proper procedure for replacing a tracheostomy tube?

_____

_____

_____

After successful replacement of the tracheostomy tube, the child's clinical condition has markedly improved. He is breathing without difficulty; his heart rate is 110 beats/min and his oxygen saturation is 97%. Breath sounds are clear and equal bilaterally. With the mother's permission, you transport to the appropriate medical facility. En route, you continue ventilations with a bag-valve-mask device, perform an ongoing assessment (**Table 19-2**), and call in your radio report to the hospital.

Table 19-2 Ongoing Assessment

Level of Consciousness	Intermittently responsive (baseline)
Airway and Breathing	Tracheostomy tube is patent; ventilations continue with a bag-valve-mask device.
Oxygen Saturation	98% (ventilated with 100% oxygen)
Blood Pressure	Not obtained
Pulse	120 beats/min, strong and regular
ECG	Normal sinus rhythm

The child is delivered to the emergency department in stable condition. You provide your verbal report to the attending physician. After additional assessment and treatment in the emergency department, the child is admitted for overnight observation and is discharged home the following day.

CASE STUDY ANSWERS AND SUMMARY

1. What is a tracheostomy? What are the indications for initial placement of a tracheostomy tube?

A tracheostomy (stoma) is a surgical opening into the trachea, just below the level of the cricoid ring (**Figure 19-1**). The tracheostomy can be used as a temporary or permanent means of providing ventilatory support to a patient.

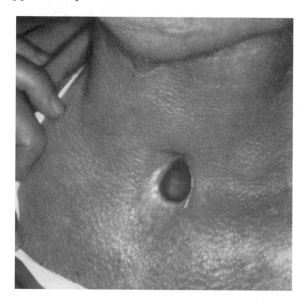

■ **Figure 19-1** A tracheostomy (stoma) is a surgical opening below the level of the cricoid ring.

A tracheostomy tube, commonly referred to as a "trach tube," is a hollow artificial airway made of plastic or metal (**Figure 19-2**). It is passed through the tracheostomy to maintain its patency and to facilitate mechanical ventilation.

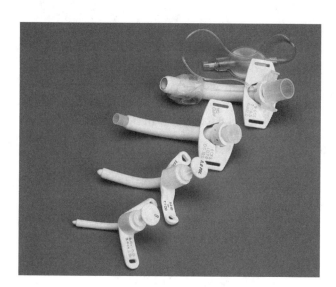

■ **Figure 19-2** Tracheostomy tubes.

There are three different types of tracheostomy tubes: fenestrated, single lumen, and double lumen (**Figure 19-3**). Tube sizes ranging from 2.5 mm to 10 mm are most commonly used in children and adolescents. Depending on the size, some tubes are equipped with a distal cuff that is filled with air to assure a tight seal; it functions the same as the distal cuff on an endotracheal tube. A proximal pilot balloon, similar to the balloon on an endotracheal tube, is present on the tracheostomy tube and serves as an indicator of whether or not the distal cuff is inflated.

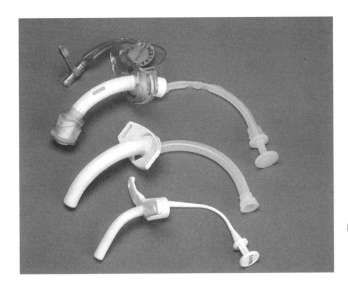

■ **Figure 19-3** Fenestrated, double lumen, and single lumen tracheostomy tubes (top to bottom).

Regardless of the type or size of the tracheostomy tube, they are all equipped with a standard 15/22-mm adaptor that connects to ventilatory devices (eg, bag-valve-mask, mechanical ventilator). Although uncommon, some tubes require an adaptor to connect to the ventilatory device. All tracheostomy tubes have an obturator, a solid plastic guide inside the tube that facilitates insertion. Because the obturator occludes the tube, it must be removed following insertion.

Single lumen tubes, which consist of one hollow tube for both airflow and suctioning of airway secretions, are most commonly used for pediatric patients. Because of the inherently small diameter of their airway, cuffed tracheostomy tubes are not used in neonates, infants, or toddlers.

A double lumen tube consists of both a hollow outer cannula and a removable hollow inner cannula. In order to provide mechanical ventilation, the inner cannula must be in place; however, it can be removed for suctioning. The additional cannula inside the double lumen tube facilitates cleaning; however, it may further decrease the tube's internal diameter, thus increasing the potential for tube obstruction by thick secretions, especially in smaller children.

A fenestrated tracheostomy tube has holes (fenestrations) that allow air to flow upward through the vocal cords and mouth. A decannulation plug is attached to the outer cannula and blocks airflow through the stoma. However, if the child is unable to breathe through the nose or mouth, this plug must be removed to allow breathing through the stoma. Unlike the single and double lumen tubes, the unique features of the fenestrated tube allow the child to talk and breathe normally with the tracheostomy tube in place.

Tracheostomy tubes are commonly placed in patients who are in need of prolonged mechanical ventilatory support. Common indications for the initial placement of a tracheostomy tube include the following:

■ **Bypassing an obstruction in the upper airway**
   • Trauma
   • Surgery
   • Congenital defects
   • Tracheal stenosis
■ **Impaired ability to clear airway secretions**

- **Need for prolonged mechanical ventilation**
  - Chronic disease processes
    - Bronchopulmonary dysplasia
    - Muscular dystrophy
  - Central nervous system deficits
    - Spinal cord injury
    - Traumatic brain injury

2. What is your next course of action?

Parents of technology-assisted children (TAC) are usually familiar with the equipment used to treat their children; they work with these devices every single day. However, despite familiarization with the equipment, some parents panic when a problem occurs. Although some paramedics may be familiar with certain types of home ventilators, this is not a regular part of their training. Additionally, this child's clinical deterioration requires prompt corrective action. Therefore, you should immediately disconnect the child from the mechanical ventilator, attach a bag-valve-mask device (without the mask, of course) to the tracheostomy tube, and begin ventilations (**Figure 19-4**). Doing so will immediately eliminate the ventilator as a possible cause of the child's respiratory distress and will allow you to continue with your assessment, perform other interventions, and, if the ventilator is not the cause of the problem, search for other possible causes.

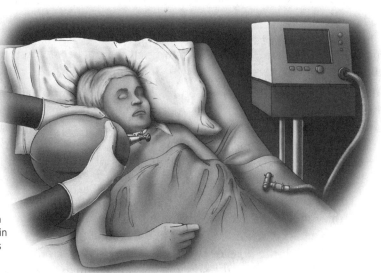

- **Figure 19-4**
Remove the child from the ventilator and begin immediate ventilations with a BVM.

3. What are the most common causes of respiratory distress in children with tracheostomy tubes? How should you proceed with your assessment?

This child's condition is clearly not improving; he is still laboring to breathe and his oxygen saturation and heart rate are decreasing. Remember, bradycardia in children with respiratory distress is an ominous sign and indicates impending respiratory or cardiopulmonary arrest. Therefore, you must act quickly to determine the underlying cause of this child's problem in order to avoid a potential disaster.

The most common causes of acute respiratory distress or failure in children who have tracheostomy tubes and are being mechanically ventilated include obstruction of the tube with secretions, inadvertent tube dislodgement, and malfunction of the mechanical ventilator. Therefore, your assessment, at least initially, should focus on these areas. Recall the DOPE mnemonic when ruling out potentially reversible causes of acute respiratory distress in the child who is being mechanically ventilated (**Table 19-3**).

Table 19-3 Assessing a Mechanically Ventilated Child Using the DOPE Mnemonic

Displacement (dislodgement) of the tube or disconnection of the tubing from the mechanical ventilator

Obstruction of airflow
- Obstruction of the tracheostomy tube
- Kinked or obstructed ventilator tubing

Pneumothorax
- Assess breath sounds to determine if they are present and equal bilaterally.

Equipment failure
- Depleted or disconnected oxygen supply
- Mechanical ventilator malfunction or failure

A crucial part of your assessment is to determine the onset and duration of the child's respiratory distress. An acute onset of respiratory distress in a child who was previously stable suggests a mechanical problem, whereas a child with progressive respiratory distress suggests an exacerbation of his or her underlying condition or a respiratory infection. Suspect a respiratory infection in a mechanically ventilated child who presents with a progressive onset of respiratory distress, fever, and adventitious (abnormal) breath sounds (eg, rales, rhonchi).

Despite removing the child from the mechanical ventilator and resuming ventilations with a bag-valve-mask device, this child's condition has not improved; therefore, ventilator malfunction is likely not the cause of his respiratory distress.

Although the child's mother has suctioned his tracheostomy tube, you should still consider tube obstruction as a possible cause of his respiratory distress. When attempting to clear an obstructed tracheostomy tube, position the child's head appropriately and ensure that the tube is in the proper position; the flange of the tube should be against the neck and the obturator should not be in place. If the child has a fenestrated tube, remove the decannulation plug. If these maneuvers are unsuccessful, the tracheostomy tube should be suctioned.

Usually, the caregiver will have the appropriate supplies and equipment available for tracheostomy suctioning. If not, select a suction catheter that is small enough to pass through the tracheostomy tube. Next, set your (or the parent's) mechanical suction device to 100 mm Hg or less. After removing the ventilatory device from the tracheostomy tube, instill 1 to 2 mL of normal saline into the tube to loosen any secretions; consider administering free-flow oxygen by holding oxygen tubing near the tube.

Without applying suction, insert the suction catheter approximately 2 to 3 inches into the tracheostomy tube (**Figure 19-5A**). You will know that the catheter is through the tube and into the trachea when the child begins to cough or retch. *Never force the catheter if resistance is felt.* Cover the suction port on the catheter and suction for 3 to 5 seconds in a circular motion while removing the catheter (**Figure 19-5B**). Never suction the tracheostomy tube for more than 10 seconds at a time. Monitor the child's oxygen saturation, heart rate, and skin color throughout the suctioning procedure. If bradycardia (heart rate < 100 beats/min), cyanosis, or significant oxygen desaturation occurs, stop suctioning immediately and provide ventilations with 100% oxygen.

After you have suctioned the tracheostomy tube, immediately reassess the child's respiratory effort, heart rate, and skin color. If improvement is noted, continue ventilations and prepare the child for transport. If the child's condition does not improve, resuctioning of the tracheostomy tube, as well as searching for other underlying causes of the child's problem, should be considered.

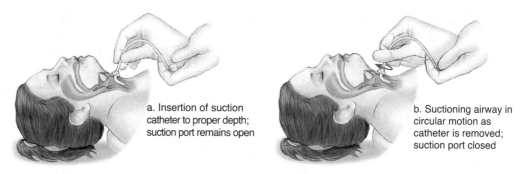

a. Insertion of suction catheter to proper depth; suction port remains open

b. Suctioning airway in circular motion as catheter is removed; suction port closed

■ **Figure 19-5** (A) Insert the suction catheter to the appropriate depth; do not suction during catheter insertion. (B) Suction the airway in a circular motion while removing the catheter.

4. What is the proper procedure for replacing a tracheostomy tube?

A tracheostomy tube must be replaced if suctioning fails to adequately clear thick secretions to allow for adequate ventilations or if decannulation (dislodgement) of the tube occurs. Although most caregivers are taught how to replace the tracheostomy tube, they may encounter problems or may not have a replacement tube available.

It is important to talk to the child and explain what you are doing, regardless of his or her mental status. If he or she is able to communicate with you, a simple explanation often facilitates the child's cooperation.

When removing the old tracheostomy tube, you may have to hyperextend the child's head to adequately expose the tracheostomy site. Apply supplemental oxygen or assist ventilations as needed and occlude the tracheostomy tube with sterile gauze and your gloved finger (**Figure 19-6**).

If the tube has a distal cuff, deflate it with a 5- or 10-mL syringe. Next, remove the cloth ties that secure the tube in place. Slowly and carefully withdraw the tube in an outward and downward motion. If needed, provide supplemental oxygen or ventilation assistance through the stoma.

If possible, you should replace the old tracheostomy tube with one of the same type and size. If the same type of tube is not available or if you are unable to reinsert the tracheostomy tube, use a similarly sized endotracheal tube.

■ **Figure 19-6**
Apply oxygen or assist ventilations as needed and occlude the tracheostomy tube.

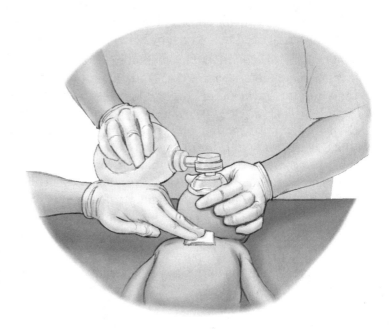

Case Study 19: Answers and Summary

If the new tube is equipped with an insertion obturator, ensure that it is placed in the tube; insert the inner cannula into the outer cannula if using a double lumen tube. Lubricate the tip of the tube and obturator with a water-soluble lubricant. Holding the tube by the flange (wings) or the tube itself like a pencil, gently but quickly insert the tube into the stoma with an arching motion (follow the curvature of the tube) posteriorly then downward. Providing slight traction above or below the stoma may facilitate insertion of the tube (**Figure 19-7**).

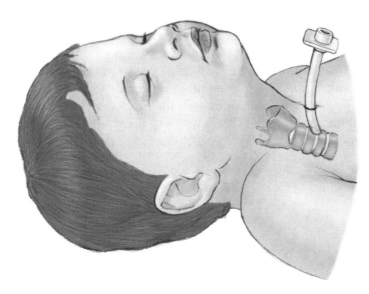

■ **Figure 19-7** Gently insert the tracheostomy tube with an arching motion, posteriorly then downward. Provide traction above or below the stoma as needed.

Never force the tube during insertion. If resistance is met, the tube may not be in the trachea; further insertion may create a false passage. After the tube is in place, remove the insertion obturator; insert the inner cannula if using a double lumen tube. Attach the ventilatory device to the tracheostomy tube and begin ventilations. Carefully stabilize the tube in place.

Confirm correct tube placement by auscultating breath sounds bilaterally, observing the chest for equal rise, and assessing the child's clinical status (eg, skin color, heart rate, oxygen saturation). Indicators of improper placement include unequal or absent breath sounds, absent chest rise, or increased resistance to ventilation. The presence of subcutaneous emphysema indicates that a false passage was created outside the trachea. If signs of improper placement are detected, immediately remove the tube and ventilate directly over the stoma. Likewise, if reinsertion of a new tracheostomy tube is unsuccessful after a few attempts, ventilate through the stoma using a protective barrier (eg, pocket mask, face shield, bag-valve-mask) or consider inserting an endotracheal tube into the stoma.

Secure the tube in place, ensuring that the tie is loose enough so that you can slide your small finger between it and the child's skin. Continue ventilations or passive oxygenation via a tracheostomy mask and transport the child to an appropriate medical facility.

Summary

Because many parents care for their chronically ill children at home, EMS personnel are responding to an increasing number of calls involving various problems with technology-assisted children (TAC). Because of this, providers must be familiar with the devices used in the management of these unique patients and must be able to troubleshoot problems if they occur. This case study depicts an acute onset of respiratory distress in a ventilator-dependent child with a permanent tracheostomy tube. Although most parents of TAC are familiar with the devices and equipment used in the treatment of their child, you may be relied upon to intervene, especially if the parent panics or is otherwise unable to rectify the situation.

Most cases of acute respiratory distress in children with tracheostomy tubes are the result of obstruction of the tube by secretions, a dislodged tube, or ventilator malfunction.

Most parents are trained to provide the appropriate interventions, including replacement of the tracheostomy tube if necessary. When caring for a child with a tracheostomy tube who experiences respiratory distress, it is important to determine the onset and duration of the problem; this will help you determine whether the underlying cause is mechanical in nature or if another problem exists, such as an exacerbation of the child's primary condition or an infection. Use the parents as your primary source of information regarding the functionality of the special equipment their child requires; they work with it every day.

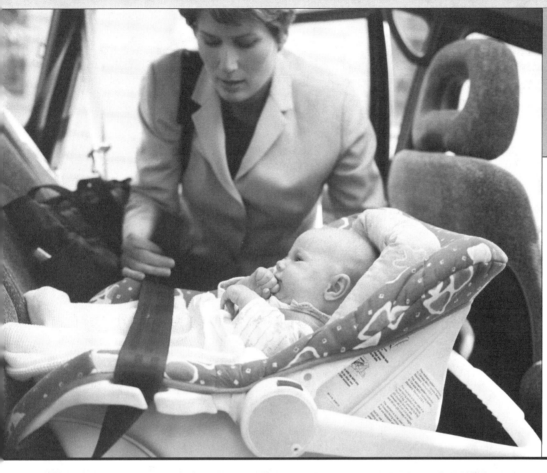

20

Childhood Injury Prevention

You have been asked to give a presentation at a Parent Teacher Association (PTA) meeting regarding childhood injury prevention. In preparation for your presentation, you research the latest data regarding the most common injuries in children and how to prevent them.

1. What is the most common cause of unintentional injury and death in children?

_____

_____

_____

You have prepared as much information as you can to disseminate to the parents and teachers. Shortly after you begin your presentation, a parent raises her hand and asks you a question regarding the proper use of child safety seats. She states that she has three children; their ages are 9 months, 3 years, and 7 years. After a brief discussion, you provide the audience with a handout that you created regarding this topic.

2. What is the appropriate method of utilizing a child safety seat?

_____

_____

_____

_____

You advise the audience that your EMS system has developed a child safety seat program, in which voluntary checkpoints are established for vehicle operators to ensure that their children are properly secured—either in a regular lap-shoulder belt or a child safety seat.

A second-grade teacher raises her hand and expresses concern regarding the number of children that she sees riding bicycles without helmets. She asks you to explain the importance of wearing helmets to the audience.

3. What information should you provide regarding the use of bicycle helmets?

_____

_____

_____

_____

After passing along some rather impressive data and statistics regarding bicycle-related deaths and how they could have been prevented by the simple use of a helmet, it is clear that you have opened quite a few eyes of your intently listening audience. The subject then turns to firearms and unintentional shootings. Many of the parents in the audience state that they have firearms in their homes and have questions about the best safety precautions to take.

4. How should you address the issue of firearm safety?

_____

_____

_____

_____

The principal of the school raises her hand and asks you if you think that their playground is safe. She states that, although a relatively small number of children have been injured on the playground, she wants to ensure that the school is following all safety precautions available.

5. What are the attributes of a "safe" playground?

_____

_____

_____

_____

Following your presentation, you receive an overwhelming round of applause from the audience. Personally, you feel that you have made an important contribution to the community and to the children who live in it.

1. What is the most common cause of unintentional injury and death in children?

According to the National Center for Injury Prevention and Control (NCIPC), motor-vehicle-related traumatic injuries account for nearly half of all unintentional pediatric injuries and deaths annually. In 2003, nearly 1,600 children between 0 and 14 years of age died as occupants in motor-vehicle crashes (MVCs); another 220,000 were injured. On average, that's four deaths and 602 injuries every day!

The two most common contributing factors to MVC-related deaths in children are failure to restrain (or properly restrain) the child and the concomitant use of alcohol by the driver. The following statistics were obtained from the National Highway Traffic Safety Administration (NHTSA):

- Of the children between 0 and 14 years of age who were killed in MVCs in 2003, more than half were unrestrained.
  - 35% of children less than 4 years of age who died in MVCs in 2003 were unrestrained.

The use of restraints or child safety seats often depends on whether or not the driver of the vehicle is restrained. Nearly 40% of children riding with drivers who are unrestrained are unrestrained themselves. Furthermore, many children who are placed in child safety seats are improperly secured. One study of more than 17,500 children riding in child safety seats revealed that only 15% were properly secured in the device.

Approximately 25% of deaths among children ages 0 to 14 years are associated with a driver under the influence of alcohol; more than two-thirds of these fatally injured children were in the same vehicle as the intoxicated driver.

2. What is the appropriate method of utilizing a child safety seat?

First, you should reinforce to the parent that how the children are secured in the vehicle may be just as important as external factors such as vehicular speed and road conditions. You should also emphasize that riding unrestrained is the *single greatest risk factor* for injury and death among children during a motor-vehicle crash.

An estimated 85% of children placed in child safety seats and booster seats are improperly secured. Following are some examples of *improperly* securing of a child in a safety seat:

- Using an inappropriate seat for the child's age and size
- Placing an infant less than 1 year of age or less than 20 pounds in a forward-facing position
- Not properly securing the safety seat in the vehicle
- Not properly securing the child in the safety seat

The safest place for a child less than 12 years of age to be when riding in a car is in the back seat. According the National Safe Kids Campaign, it is estimated that children ages 12 years and younger are nearly 40% less likely to die in a motor-vehicle crash if they are in the rear seat of a passenger vehicle.

The following recommendations regarding child passenger safety were obtained from the American Academy of Pediatrics (AAP), the Centers for Disease Control and Prevention (CDC), and the National Highway Traffic Safety Administration (NHTSA):

- Until a child is at least 1 year of age or at least 20 pounds (9 kg), he or she should ride in the back seat of a passenger vehicle and should be secured in a rear-facing infant seat.

- Convertible seats can be used in children less than 1 year of age or less than 20 pounds provided the seat is placed in a reclined and rear-facing position.
  - NEVER place a rear-facing safety seat (standard or convertible) in the front passenger seat of a vehicle equipped with a passenger-side airbag.
- Children who are older than 1 year of age and weigh more than 20 to 40 pounds (9 to 18 kg) can be placed in a convertible safety seat used in an upright, forward-facing position.
  - The child must fit well in the safety seat.
  - The harness straps should be positioned at or above the child's shoulders.
  - The seat should be placed in the back seat of the passenger vehicle.
- Child booster seats should be used for children who weigh between 40 and 80 pounds (18 to 36 kg) or until they are at least 4'10" tall.
  - Booster seats ensure that the lap and shoulder belts restrain the child over bony areas, rather than areas of soft tissue.
  - The lap belt should be low and snugly fastened across the child's hips; the shoulder harness should cross from the child's clavicles across the sternum to the hip. *The shoulder harness must not cross the child's neck.*

A child can be placed in a regular seatbelt *when the belt fits properly*. This means that the shoulder harness must lie across the middle of the chest and shoulder, not the neck or throat; the lap belt should be low and snug across the hips, not the abdomen. Additionally, the child's legs should be long enough so the knees bend at the edge of the seat. Remember, seatbelts are designed for adults. If the seatbelt does not fit the child correctly, he or she should remain in a booster seat. Most children can be safely secured in a regular seatbelt when they reach about 4'10" tall and are between 8 and 12 years of age.

Remember, however, that no child under 12 years of age should ride in the front seat of an automobile, especially if it is equipped with passenger-side airbags. The National Safe Kids Campaign reported that, as of January 1, 2004, 141 children have been killed by passenger-side airbags. Furthermore, many of these children were either unrestrained or improperly restrained at the time of impact.

You should advise parents that the manufacturer of their automobile may have specific requirements relating to the use of restraint seats/systems that are unique to that particular make and model of automobile (eg, specific seat fixation points).

3. What information should you provide regarding the use of bicycle helmets?
First of all, this teacher has every right to be concerned; many children don't wear helmets when riding their bicycles. In fact, national estimates report that helmet use among child bicyclists ranges from about 15% to 25%; it is lowest in children between the ages of 11 to 14 years. Common excuses include:

- It's too uncomfortable.
- I'm a good bike rider.
- I look like a "geek."
- None of my friends wear helmets.

More than 70% of children between the ages of 5 and 14 years ride bicycles. This same age group also rides about 50% more than the average bicyclist. Therefore, it is no surprise that approximately one quarter of all bicycle-related deaths and more than half of all bicycle-related injuries occur in children between 5 and 14 years of age.

Bicycles are second only to the automobile, in terms of childhood injuries caused. In 2001, 134 children under 14 years of age died in bicycle-related incidents; in 2002, nearly 290,000 children were treated in emergency departments for bicycle-related injuries.

Head injury is the leading cause of death secondary to bicycle crashes and is the most important determinant of permanent disability. For obvious reasons, the single most effective way to reduce the risk of experiencing a head injury from a bicycle crash is to wear a helmet. In fact, wearing a helmet can reduce the risk of head injury by as much as 85%! Children who do not wear helmets are 14 times more likely to experience fatal injuries following a bicycle crash than riders who wear helmets. It is estimated that 75% of bicycle-related deaths among children could have been prevented if a helmet were worn.

So, how do you know which bicycle helmet is most appropriate for your child? First, you should buy a helmet that meets or exceeds current safety standards; these helmets will have a sticker from one of the following organizations:

- U.S. Consumer Product Safety Commission (CPSC)
- American National Standards Institute (ANSI)
- American Society for Testing and Materials (ASTM)
- Snell Helmet Safety Standards

The helmet should sit on top of your child's head in a level position. It should cover his or her forehead and not rock back and forth or from side to side. The child in **Figure 20-1** is *not* wearing her helmet properly; it is positioned too far back on her head, exposing her forehead to injury. To ensure that you select the correct size, perform the "Eyes, Ears, and Mouth" check (**Table 20-1**).

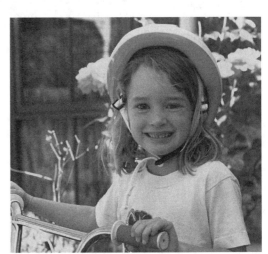

- **Figure 20-1** As worn, this helmet would not protect the child's forehead from injury.

Table 20-1 The Ears, Eyes, and Mouth Check of Helmet Sizing

Eyes	
• Position the helmet on the child's head. Look up and you should see the bottom rim of the helmet, one to two fingers above the eyebrows.	
Ears	
• Ensure that the straps of the helmet form a "V" under the child's ears when buckled. The strap should be snug but comfortable.	
Mouth	
• Ask your child to open his or her mouth as wide as possible; if he or she cannot feel the helmet "hug" his or her head, the straps need to be tightened.	

Currently, 19 states and the District of Columbia—as well as numerous localities—have enacted some form of bicycle helmet legislation, most of which pertain to children. It is important for you to be familiar with the laws and regulations of your locale or state.

The National Safe Kids Campaign has identified the following additional risk factors that contribute to death and disability in children who ride bicycles:

- Approximately 60% of fatal bicycle crashes occur at nonintersection locations; 80% of these crashes occur between the months of April and October; 65% occur between the hours of 2:00 PM and 8:00 PM.
- Children are four times more likely to be injured or killed when riding at night, dawn, or dusk than those who ride in daylight.
- Children are more likely to experience injury or death when riding on residential streets close to home; many deaths occur within 1 mile of the child's residence.
- Approximately 60% of all childhood bicycle-related deaths occur on minor roads.
- Children under 4 years of age are more likely than older children to be injured around the home (eg, driveway, garage).

A child's riding behavior is also a significant risk factor. Most bicycle-related deaths occur when children enter a street without stopping first, or are turning left or swerving into traffic coming from behind, running a stop sign, or riding against the flow of traffic. Bicycle collisions with motor vehicles account for nearly 90% of all bicycle-related deaths.

It is important for both children and their parents to realize that a bicycle is a vehicle, not a toy. Like any other vehicle, there are certain "rules of the road" that should be learned and practiced on a regular basis. Parents should teach their children the following:

- Ride with the flow of traffic, not against it.
- Ride as far to the right of traffic as possible.
- Use appropriate hand signals.
- Respect traffic signals; stop at all red lights and stop signs.
- When entering a street; stop and look left, right, and then left again.
- Before turning left at an intersection, look back and yield to traffic approaching from the rear.
- Don't ride when it's dark. If riding at dusk, dawn, or night is unavoidable, wear a reflective vest and use lights and reflectors on the bike.
- Simply put—no helmet, no bike!

Children under 10 years of age should not be allowed to ride their bike to school. Even for children older than 10 years of age, the parent should determine if the child has mastered the essential traffic skills that come with riding a bike.

Whether the path to school involves riding on the street or not, parents should take the time to plan a safe bicycle route with their children and should ride it with them. Bear in mind, however, that the safest cycling route may be different from the safest walking route.

4. How should you address the issue of firearm safety?

Some parents believe their children are safe because there are no firearms in their home; others believe their children are safe because they do have firearms in the home and their children are aware of "the rules." The reality is that *all* children are potentially at risk of unintentional injury from firearms.

Nearly two thirds of parents who own firearms and have school-age children believe that they keep the firearm stored safely away, out of reach of their children. One study, however, indicated that 75% to 80% of first- and second-graders indeed knew where it was kept.

While most children over 8 years of age can reliably distinguish between a real gun and a toy gun, they do not fully understand the capabilities of a firearm. Frighteningly, children as young as 3 years of age are strong enough to pull the trigger of many handguns.

Most unintentional shooting deaths occur in or around the home; 50% of deaths occur in the child's home and nearly 40% occur at the home of a friend or relative. The vast majority of these deaths involved guns that were kept loaded and improperly secured. One study of parents with children who ranged in age from 4 to 12 years found that more than 50% admitted to storing a firearm—loaded or improperly secured—in their home. An estimated 3.3 million children in the United States live in homes with firearms that are always or sometimes kept loaded and/or improperly secured.

In 2002, approximately 800 children under 14 years of age required treatment in the emergency department for unintentional firearm injuries; in 2001, 72 children were killed as a result of unintentional shootings.

The following risk factors for unintentional firearm injuries have been identified by the National Safe Kids Campaign:

- **Most shootings occur when children are unsupervised and out of school.**
  - Most unintentional shootings occur between 4:00 PM and 5:00 PM, during the weekends, and during the summer months.

- **Unintentional firearm incidents are higher in rural areas, where people are more likely to own firearms; shotguns or rifles are the most commonly involved firearms.**
  - In cities, handguns are the most commonly involved firearm; most incidents occur indoors.

- **Males are more likely to be injured or killed as a result of firearm-related injuries than females. In fact, nearly 85% of children killed by unintentional shootings are males.**

Firearms are kept in homes for two reasons: protection or sport. Unfortunately, if used for protection, a gun is useless if it's locked up in the closet. Therefore, it is absolutely critical to educate children regarding firearm safety. Many parents take their children to a shooting range and allow them to actually shoot the gun. By demonstrating what the gun is capable of doing (eg, blasting a target or other object to bits), the child will likely garner a healthy appreciation and respect for firearms. Remember, unintentional shootings occur because of a lack of understanding.

If the firearm is not used for protection purposes, it has no business in the drawer next to your bed! **Table 20-2** summarizes the precautions that all gun owners who have children should take; **Table 20-3** summarizes precautions that all parents should take, even if they do not own a firearm.

Table 20-2 Safety Precautions for Gun Owners with Children

Store all firearms unloaded, locked up, and out of reach of all children in the home.
Store all ammunition in a separate, locked-up location.
If possible, store all firearms in a gun safe, lock box, or other container that is inaccessible to the child. • Keep all keys and combinations to safes or lock boxes with firearms hidden in a separate location.
Educate your child regarding the appropriate use, safety, and storage of firearms. • If the child is old enough, have him or her take a course in firearm safety.

Table 20-3 Safety Precautions for All Parents

Educate children regarding the danger associated with firearms.
Teach children never to touch or play with a gun.
Teach children to tell an adult or call 9-1-1 if they find a gun.
Check with neighbors, friends, and relatives—or adults in any other homes where children visit—to ensure that they safely store their firearms, if they own any.

Remember, children are inherently curious. If they are not properly educated regarding firearms, they will attempt to educate themselves. Unfortunately, this usually involves looking *and* touching without knowledge of the weapon's capabilities. It should be reiterated that parents should educate their children about firearms, even if they do not own a gun. Remember, many unintentional firearm-related deaths occur when the child is visiting a friend's house, where the parents do own firearms.

5. What are the attributes of a "safe" playground?

More than 53 million American children spend nearly one fourth of their waking lives in school or on school property. As a result, an estimated 10% to 25% of the more than 14 million unintentional injuries experienced by children annually occur in and around schools. A significant portion of these injuries occur on playgrounds; others occur during physical education (PE) classes, organized sports activities, and around school buses.

Playground injuries are the most common school-related injuries in children between 5 and 14 years of age. Eighty percent of the most serious playground injuries—head injuries and fractures—are the result of falls. The risk of injury is four times greater if the child falls from an object that is more than 5′ in height. Clearly, young children who play on equipment designed for older children are at increased risk for injury.

More than 50% of playground equipment-related deaths are attributed to strangulation injuries, such as when the child's clothing becomes tangled or he or she is trapped in various playground equipment.

Regardless of the mechanism of playground injury, children are more likely to be injured when they are not supervised by an adult. Lack of adult supervision is associated with approximately 40% of playground-related injuries.

As with any other activity discussed in this case study, education is the key to prevent injuries in children while they are at school. Parents should teach their children not to push, shove, or crowd when on the playground. Children should be taught to differentiate between equipment that is and is not appropriate for their age.

So, what are the attributes of a "safe" playground? The safest playgrounds are well-maintained (no broken, protruding, or loose parts) and should have ample surfacing, such as mulch chips, pea gravel, fine sand, or shredded rubber (**Figure 20-2**). Playgrounds with asphalt, concrete, grass, or soil surfaces should be avoided. The playground surface should be at least 12″ deep and should extend a minimum of 6 feet in all directions surrounding stationary equipment.

Regardless of the safety of the playground, there must be adequate adult supervision for the number of children on the playground at any one time. Additionally, teachers should ensure that children only play on equipment that is appropriate for their age. There should be separate playgrounds for children of various ages.

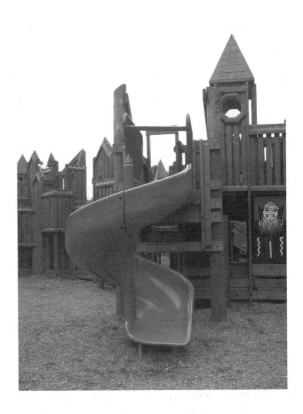

■ **Figure 20-2** Soft or absorbent surfaces on playgrounds will significantly decrease the risk of serious injury if a child falls.

Summary

Despite appropriate prehospital care and rapid transport to an appropriate medical facility, a significant number of children die every year as the result of unintentional injuries. As EMS personnel, we are consequence managers; our services are not needed until the injury has occurred. Clearly, taking steps to prevent injuries in the first place can have a profound impact on the safety of our children.

Injuries, whether intentional or unintentional, are often predictable based on the study of injury patterns. Like certain illnesses, injuries often vary with the seasons, may occur epidemically, and often follow demographic distributions. If injuries are predictable as to how and when they occur, they are potentially preventable as well. Whether providing "on the spot" education to the parent of a non–critically-injured child or offering formal injury prevention programs, the EMS community has a responsibility to educate the public regarding a wide array of childhood injury prevention strategies. Those discussed in this case study—albeit the most common—are just a few strategies.

Note: Statistical data cited in this case study were obtained from the following resources and were current as of April 3, 2005:

- **Centers for Disease Control and Prevention:** *www.cdc.gov*
- **National Center for Injury Prevention and Control:** *www.cdc.gov/ncipc/default.htm*
- **National Safe Kids Campaign:** *www.safekids.org*
- **National Highway Traffic Safety Administration:** *www.nhtsa.dot.gov*
- **American Academy of Pediatrics:** *www.aap.org*
- **EMS for Children:** *www.ems-c.org*

ADDITIONAL CREDITS

Chapter 2
Opener; 2-2: Courtesy of Ronald A. Deickmann, MD

Chapter 3
Opener: Courtesy of David J. Burchfield, MD

Chapter 4
Opener: © Eddie Sperling

Chapter 6
Opener: © Adam Gault/Digital Vision/Getty Images

Chapter 8
Opener: © Merrill Dyck/ShutterStock, Inc.
8-2: Courtesy of Ronald A. Deickmann, MD

Chapter 9
Opener: Courtesy of the National EMSC Slideset

Chapter 10
Opener: © Perry Correll/ShutterStock, Inc.

Chapter 13
13-4: Courtesy of Marianne Gausche-Hill, MD

Chapter 16
Opener: Courtesy of Marianne Gausche-Hill, MD

Chapter 17
Opener: Used with permission of the American Academy of Pediatrics, *APLS: The Pediatric Emergency Medicine Resource*, 4th Edition, American Academy of Pediatrics and American College of Emergency Physicians, 2004.

17-1; 17-2; 17-3: Used with permission of the American Academy of Pediatrics, *Pediatric Education for Prehospital Providers*, American Academy of Pediatrics, 2000.

Chapter 18
18-1: © Mediscan/Visuals Unlimited

18-2: Courtesy of the Centers for Disease Control

Chapter 19
Opener; 19-1: Courtesy of Marianne Gausche-Hill, MD

Chapter 20
Opener: © Ryan McVay/Photodisc/Getty Images

20-1; 20-2: Courtesy of Ronald A. Deickmann, MD

Rhythm strips throughout the text are from *Arrhythmia Recognition: The Art of Interpretation*, courtesy of Tomas B. Garcia, MD.

Unless otherwise indicated, photographs and illustrations are supplied by Jones and Bartlett Publishers.